Those of us who have received an organ transplant are forever grateful to our donor and their family

A QUEST FOR A LUNG

A Journey Through Transplant

By
Ron Chapman

Other Books by this Author

But for a Piece of Wood: The Battle of New Orleans

Louisiana: A Journey Through Time

Is St. Bernard Doomed?

Chalmette Refining:100 Years

Another Day in Paradise: A Katrina Story

Battle of New Orleans Reconsidered (contributed)

Crime and Punishment in Lower Norfolk County, Virginia 1637-1676

(Master's Thesis)

In Memory of a Dear Friend

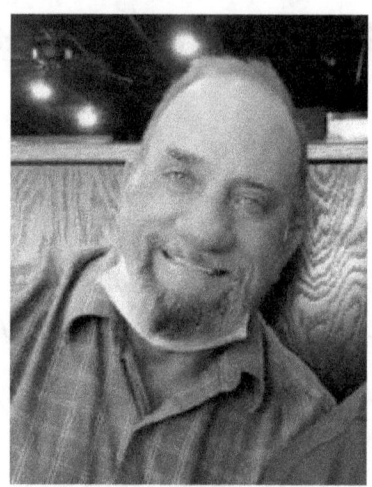

Mike Tredinich

*Met Mike and his wife Janet at Nora Home.
Wonderful people and good friends. We will miss
him greatly. He was my mentor on this shared
journey. We miss his smile and insights.*

Special Thanks

I am forever grateful to my lovely wife Margaret, my daughter Becca, and to her husband Calvin Kia Ku. They have been such champions for me and provided the support required. Many do not realize the level of personal commitment required to become a Care Giver.

I also wish to thank Charles and Claudette Ponstein, my brother-in-law and sister-in-law, for maintaining the home front in our absence. Such relief during this long ordeal.

Additionally, it is critical to acknowledge all of my friends and colleagues who did everything in their power to make this Quest possible. I could not have done it without them.

In a final note, how can one not provide special thanks to the Houston Methodist Hospital Pulmonary Team that gave me this "new lease on life", because that is indeed what it is. The level of professionalism on all levels is inspiring. They are indeed miracle workers.

Last but certainly not least, is Dr. Joseph Lasky and his team at Tulane Medical. Iris Manuel, Sandy Ditta, and Jennifer Fitzgibbons are amazing and caring people. Were it not for them I would not be here, nor would I have been sent to Houston Methodist for transplant.

Ron Chapman

Very Special Thanks to the Doctors, Nurses, and Staff of Houston Methodist Hospital. They gave me the gift of life for which I am forever thankful.

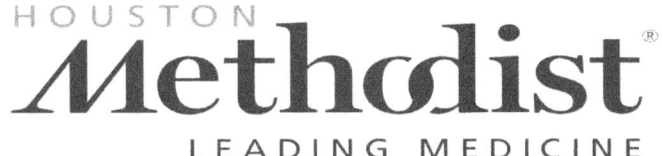

Contents

Reflections

Ours has been an interesting journey, but not just a medical one. It runs far deeper. Housing is limited to ninety days. We move from one place to another in three-month cycles. As a result, we have the occasion to meet so many different people, with different backgrounds, different ethnicities, different ages, and different medical challenges.

Few people travel the transplant road, but perhaps more than we think. Some of you reading this now may find yourselves walking this path in the future. It opens one's eyes to aspects of life and the struggle for survival a few people experience.

I have witnessed the sorrow of someone's passing. Of patients being rejected for treatment, I was one of those myself. I have witnessed success, as I have experienced as well. Both are sides of the same coin. The stories are about young and old. But in all cases, it is a story of courage, dedication, compassion, love and too often resignation to fate.

This is a private world. Set aside from the daily adventures of the rest of society. An all-encompassing world where the thoughts that trouble most do not intrude. Because in this world only one thing matters...survival.

It is not like going to a doctor, getting a shot, and getting better. Were that it was so. No, this world is one of persistent focus. It is an existence tied to routine and medications. A world subject to sudden changes. A world where one never knows if tomorrow things might change for *the better or worse. You experience the intensity of life on a knife's edge.*

Nevertheless, it is not a depressing world. Quite the contrary. This existence stays focused on living every day to its extreme. Here clarity reigns because that which is important becomes abundantly clear. One knows what matters most.

The general population wakes up every morning thinking about what is important for that day. Like a test tube with thoughts and troubles mixed within the fluid. They open the top of the container and what floats to the surface is what they believe matters. In our world, that same test tube is placed in a centrifuge and spun. What truly matters comes to the top and those considerations of truly less importance fall to the bottom...as sediment.

You know life is short because most likely you have already measured it at least once. One starts seriously reflecting on life and its meaning. Everyday concerns fall by the wayside as you strive to find meaning and purpose for the time remaining.

This is not a sad journey. It can be most enlightening in so many ways. You learn about people, sacrifice, love, dedication, professionalism, science, and most importantly how to trust those around you who have placed your interests above all others. You learn humility and the strength of the human spirit to overcome adversity.

Although it can be long, measured in years, and arduous, it is also rewarding. The bonds and friendships you create with your fellow travelers are unbreakable. Everyone is giving. This is how the world should be.

Thus, despite the hardships that come with the voyage, the voyage itself is rewarding in immeasurable ways. I certainly do not wish this on anyone. However, if you find yourself on this path, take heed and open your eyes. You are not alone and will be experiencing a facet of life few know about. Embrace it.

No matter how the final destination unfolds, the journey itself is enlightening and rewarding in so many ways. You will develop a much deeper understanding of the world about you and the people who populate it.

Ron

Introduction

You are about to take a journey. The quest for lungs is complicated and long. From the moment of diagnosis of a serious lung disease, one must realize that the only way to stay alive is to gain a transplant. Knowing that should drive your every effort to achieve that goal.

By the time I received my transplant, I was using 9.5 liters of oxygen per minute sitting down and 25 Liters when I attempted to do anything! I was at *"end stage interstitial lung disease."* My diagnosis was Hypersensitivity Pneumonitis which evolved into IPF (Idiopathic Pulmonary Fibrosis).

The following is a guide to help you along your path. There are many issues with which you will have to contend. Your health comes first, followed by social, economic, emotional, and housing. This is intended to help educate you about what you must learn to ease the way through this endeavor.

I am a 74-year-old male in generally good health other than being initially "Unclassified" as regards to the nature and origin of my Interstitial Lung Disease (ILD). When diagnosed I realized that my and my family's life suddenly changed. My age created problems, I was considered "High Risk" based solely on my number of "trips around the Sun", where age is truly driven by DNA and state of mind. Nevertheless, because of several miracles, I was able to be transplanted.

My sole intention throughout was to stay alive and that motivated my every move. This short work seeks to provide a guidebook for those similarly afflicted. The basic process of qualification for lung transplant is the same for everyone no matter the organ involved. What I discovered though was despite the commonness of the venture, there were no guides to the overall process. One had to figure things out for themselves. That motivated e to compose this short book

Yes, indeed there are some splendid works like "Exhale" by Doctor David Weill. He gives readers an excellent insight into the transplant process as well as being a "must read" for anyone on the quest. But there was still very little work informing patients about the tangled web one must traverse on a personal level.

This work seeks to deliver insights into the process one must follow, and the preparations needed in the most practical sense…how to navigate the journey. My personal story illustrates my process, my struggles, and my success (thus far).

Special thanks to Dr. Janine Parker, my initial pulmonologist. To Dr. Joseph Lasky of Tulane Medical School, the pulmonologist she referred me to because of the difficulty in assessing my case. Dr. Joseph Lasky is an amazing doctor and has become a special friend. He made the referrals for transplant.

However, I owe special appreciation to the Doctors and Staff of Houston's Methodist Hospital Pulmonary Department, I would not be here were it not for them.

At Methodist Hospital there are far too many dedicated practitioners to mention, and I hate to miss anyone. That being said, I owe the following individuals a deep debt of gratitude: Dr. Howard Huang (Chief of Lung Transplantation), Dr. Sandeep Sahay (Pulmonologist), Dr. J Georges Youssef (Pulmonologist), Dr. Mea Botros (Pulmonary Critical Care), Dr. Ahmed Goodarzi (Pulmonary), Dr. Joggy Georges (Cardiologist), Dr. Simon Yau (Pulmonologist), Dr. Steven Koch (Critical Care), Dr. Erik Suarez (Surgical Director), Jennifer Hguyen FNP (Epidemiology), and Uy Ngo PA who brightens every room he enters. Special regards to Manju Johns, my Transplant Coordinator who is always there to help. They all deserve accolades. They are the master players of my experience… my transplant team.

I would be remiss if I did not mention the fine care I received at Baylor St. Lukes where my initial testing was performed. Even though I was eventually denied transplant, Dr. Puneet Garcha and Gabriel Loor deserve my admiration for their efforts and the help they provided in the early stages of my journey.

For all of these doctors, nurses, and staff, I have nothing but respect and love. They made a very harrowing experience less stressful because of their dedication, patient care, and general respect for one another. My experience at Houston Methodist turned my life around because of their efforts. For that I am forever grateful to everyone. Houston Methodist is an amazing hospital with modern equipment and is a wonderful facility. But it is the people that make it so special. They perform truly as a team in the grandest sense of the word.

The Quest for Lungs" presents many challenges, but having true professionals as guides and practitioners eases the journey.

Again, I will pay homage to my wife Margaret, my daughter Becca, her husband Calvin Kia Ku, and the rest of my family, friends, and colleagues who provided the necessary support for success. It could not have been achieved without their love and care. You cannot succeed without support. This network made everything possible. I love them all "To the Moon and Back."

The slogan I espoused throughout was "All Will Be Well!" My chancellor, Dr. Tina Tinney, at Nunez Community College where I work as a Professor of History provided that insight when she brought me a medal early in this venture. That has become my slogan ever since.

This said, the Quest begins…

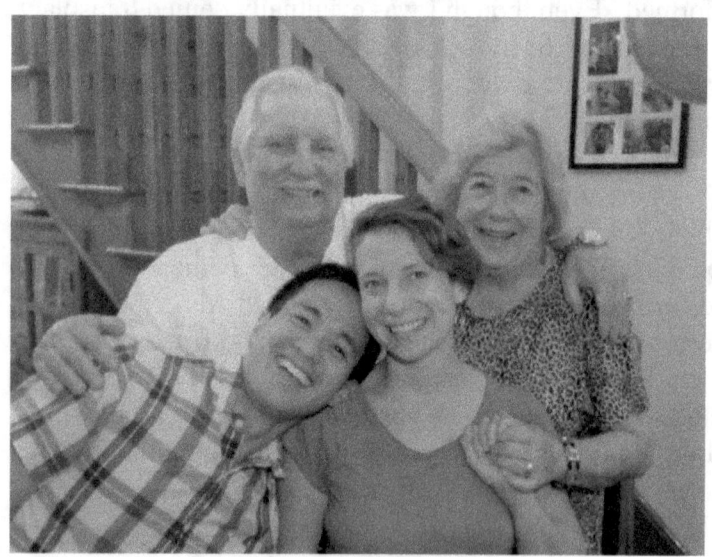

Calvin, Becca, Margaret, & Ron

A QUEST FOR A LUNG

This brief guide focuses on the journey that has been thrust upon you. It should help in understanding your path. Though not welcomed, nevertheless, it is now a part of your life. Accept reality and never allow yourself to wallow in sorrow. That is not a healthy state of mind. You must be strong to prevail, and you will prevail if you are determined to survive. So much depends upon attitude, so develop a good one if it alludes you now.

When you are diagnosed with a chronic lung disease like Cystic Fibrosis (CF), Idiopathic Pulmonary Fibrosis (IPF), Hypersensitivity Pneumonitis (HP), or Usual Interstitial Pneumonia (IUP), your life changes. The regular challenges of life fall to the background. Your total focus becomes a mission to "breathe." You will likely be facing a lung transplant.

Your family and friends will be devastated by the news. Expect some emotions. You will need support. Start now to build that support base. The ready availability of several very dependable and close family members and friends who are willing to take on the burden is essential. It WILL be a burden sometimes. They may never state it, but the impositions on time and energy can be daunting. Members of the support team must become aware of this from the onset because you will need them long-term. This is a marathon, not a sprint. YOU *HAVE TO ASK FOR HELP.*

As your condition gets worse, they will be called upon to take you to doctors' visits, hospital appointments for testing, and other perhaps mundane but necessary tasks like grocery shopping. A dependable network is essential, especially as one approaches needing a transplant.

Initially, while the disease is mild, it will not inhibit your life. Later, as your symptoms become more pronounced, your lifestyle will become limited. At first, oxygen may only be required for sleep. Later you will be using a low dose which can be achieved by means of a portable unit. Eventually, your breathing limitations will require a larger Oxygen Concentrator which is not portable. This means being restricted to your home.

As you approach end stage, you will find yourself being totally confined to your home, with a few exceptions, on oxygen 24/7. As I always commented: I could do anything I wish as long as it was within a 30-foot radius…hose length! Your ability to emotionally adjust to using oxygen determines this phase.

Having hobbies proves an advantage. Your physical activities are limited. When homebound, it can play on your mind, especially if you have nothing to do while at home. Any interest you have like reading, painting, writing or whatever can be a mental health savior. This gives you something to wake up for and be excited about. Otherwise, you may find yourself lost in depression. Just sitting in a recliner and watching TV is not conducive to a positive attitude. That is not healthy.

If you do not have a hobby, find one! You may be surprised to discover a talent you never knew you had. This is all a part of keeping a necessary positive attitude. Your approach to this new challenge is critical. The doctors gauge this very seriously.

You must overcome any embarrassment you may encounter about public use of oxygen. This can be difficult; it was for me. It is somehow a public admission of weakness and illness. Get over it. Otherwise, you will miss out on too many important experiences. The time will come too soon when you will not be able to go out because of the quantity of oxygen needed. Most portable battery units supply only 3 liters max on pulse. (More on that later). So, make the best of the time and mobility you have while you have it.

The status of your disease will determine the course of action taken by you and your pulmonologist. There are numerous treatments available that might slow down the process (Esbriet, OFEV, Tyvaso, and now Jascayd), but generally a steady decline in breathing can be expected. That requires constant adjustments to your situation.

Your doctor will likely prescribe Oxygen Therapy. This will be prescribed as a result of a six-minute walk. Insurance usually covers this expense. However, the coverage is limited. If you have a second home you spend time in, you will have to purchase a second concentrator yourself. This is easy to do, and they are home delivered from an online store in a matter of days. You will need a prescription. It may cost about $600-$1,000 depending on the size. I purchased a 10 liter because I knew I would eventually need that much.

You have three oxygen options to consider: a portable concentrator, or a continuous flow concentrator, or a tank. Each has its benefits and limitations. A portable has limited oxygen available duration dependent on battery size. A tank has concentrated oxygen available at high levels but is heavy and short term. The concentrator is not portable but necessary for home use.

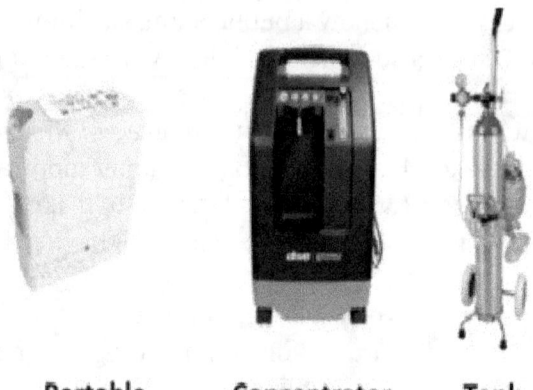

Portable   Concentrator   Tank

Oxygen concentrators come in two flavors. Pulse Activation means that oxygen is supplied when the patient inhales. This uses less oxygen and is the only method available with portable oxygen concentrators. These small units generally supply 1-3 liters per minute. The settings only apply to the size of the bolus, the specific size of the puff of oxygen you receive.

Portable units permit mobility. You can attend events, go to dinner, theater…do whatever you desire within the limits of battery power. The higher the user rate, the lower the battery life. It is suggested that you have replacement batteries on hand as a backup. They are not cheap. These portable units are pulse only. Also, check with manufacturers to see how much oxygen is actually delivered. The settings button on top of the unit is NOT the amount of oxygen delivered. It is merely a setting.

The chart below describes the different Personal Oxygen Concentrators (POC) and their data:

Brand or Manufacturer	Portable Oxygen Concentrators (POC)	POC Weight in Pounds	LPM on Highest Setting	Battery Weight	Battery Life in Hours	Change Time Hours	Watt Hours (Wh)	Decibels	Pulse Delivery Type	Customer Replace Sieve	Pulse Levels/Settings
Inogen	G4 (same as Flt)	2.8/3.3	0.63 lpm	6/1.1	2.7/5°	3/5	50.9/98.6	40**	Minute	✓	1-3
Oxygen	Flt (same as G4)	2.8/3.3	0.63 lpm	6/1.1	2.7/5°	3/5	50.9/98.6	40**	Minute	✓	1-3
Inogen	Rove 4	2.8/3.1/3.4	0.84 lpm	6/.8/1.1	9/14/18***	5/3/4	50.6/71.15/93.6	39**	Minute	✓	1-4
Rhythm	P2-S3	3.3/4/4.4	0.63 lpm	3/1/1.4	1.2/2.5/3.5***	2/4/6	49/98/147*	<45***	Minute	No	1-3
Rhythm	P2-S4 (same as Ayra Mini)	3.3/4/4.4	0.84 lpm	3/1/1.4	1/2/3****	2/4/6	49/98/147*	<45***	Minute	No	1-4
Arya	Arya Mini (same as P2-S4)	3.3/4/4.4	0.84 lpm	3/1/1.4	1/2/3****	2/4/6	49/98/147*	<45***	Minute	No	1-4
Belluscura	XPLO_R	3.29°	0.75 lpm	0.5	<= 4.5°	<= 6	92/6	<19**	Minute	✓	1-4
Rhythm	P2 (same as AirThro)	4.37	1 lpm		<2 level 3	4	98	49**	Minute	No	1-5
Arya	AirThro (same as P2)	4.37	1 lpm		<2 level 5	4	98	49**	Minute	No	1-5
Rhythm	P2-E6 (same as AirThro Max)	4.37	1.33 lpm		1.7 level 6	4	98	49**	Minute	No	1-6
Arya	AirThro Max (same as P2-E6)	4.37	1.00 lpm		1.7 level 6	4	98	49**	Minute	No	1-6
Rhythm	P2-E7	4.37	1.46 lpm		1.2 level 7	4	98	49**	Minute	No	1-7
Inogen	G5 (same as Next)	4.8/5.8	1.26 lpm	1.2/2.2	6.5°/13°	3/6	47.2+47.2/92.2+92.2°	38**	Minute	✓	1-6
OxyGo	NEXT (same as G5)	4.8/5.8	1.26 lpm	1.2/2.2	6.5°/13°	3/6	47.2+47.2/92.2+92.2°	38**	Minute	✓	1-6
Inogen	Rove 6 (similar to G5)	4.8/5.8	1.28 lpm	1.2/2.2	6.5°/13°	3/6	47.2+47.2/92.2+92.2°	39**	Minute	✓	1-6
DeVilbiss	iGo2 (seems to be same as Arya Q)	4.95	1.01 lpm	0.81	3.5**	<3	72.36	<37.5**	Minute	No	1-5
Arya	Arya Q (seems to be same as iGo2)	4.8	1.01 lpm	0.81	3.5**	<3	72.36	<41	Minute	No	1-5
Caire	FreeStyle Comfort (same as Arya Go)	5°	1.09 lpm	1.2/2.2	8°/16°	3.5/6	06.5	39.9**	Minute	No	1-5
Arya	Arya Go (same as FreeStyle Comfort)	5°	1.05 lpm	1.2/2.2	8°/16°	3.5/6	06.5	39.9**	Minute	No	1-5
Precision Medical	Live Active 5	5	1 lpm		6°		94.7	<40**	Minute	✓	1-5
GCE	Zen-O Lite (same as Arya P5)	5.5	1.09 lpm	0.97	4.5**	2.5	98.6	37**	Both	✓	1-10
Arya	Arya P5 (same as Zen-O Lite)	5.5	1.05 lpm	0.97	4.5**	2.5	98.6	37**	Both	✓	1-10
O2 Concepts	OxLife Liberty	6.30°	1.5 lpm / 1.5 @ 1.5 lpm	1.14	1.25 on level 9 / 1.5 @ 1.5 lpm	2.5	96.48	44.4**	Both	No	1-9 / 1-5
O2 Concepts	OxLife Liberty2	6.36°	14 lpm / 2 lpm	1.14	1.25 on level 10 / 1 @ 2 lpm	2.5	96.48	44.4**	Both	No	1-10 / 1-7
Belluscura	DISCOV-R	6.9°	1.5 lpm / 2 lpm	0.6	2.5**	<= 6	92/6	42.7**	Both	✓	1-5
GCE	Zen-O	10.25	2 lpm / 2 lpm	1.06	4° / 8°		96	3B / 42	Both	No	1-6 / 1-4
O2 Concepts	Independence	16.7	1.02 lpm / 3 lpm	1.4	1.76*** / 2.5 @ 2 lpm	2.5	95	56 @ 3 lpm	Fixed	No	1-6
Claire	SeQual Eclipse 5	18.4	192 lpm / 3 lpm	5.4	6.4** / 2 @ 2 lpm	1.0	88.9 + 98.9°	40** / 48 @ 3 lpm	Fixed	No	1-9 / 1-6

The constant flow oxygen concentrator is much larger and supplies oxygen at a steady rate. The oxygen continuously flows through the cannula, which is the hose that connects the oxygen unit to your nose for intake. These units come in two versions 1-5 liters per minute or 1-10 liters per minute. The latter unit is much louder than the first. Something to keep in mind. Also, sound levels differ among vendors of concentrators. Respironics 10L Millennium is very quiet.

Oxygen tanks come in a variety of sizes with varying capacities. The chart below provides some information on that score. They do provide continuous flow but as stated earlier they are heavy, awkward, and short term. They do, however, serve a purpose. If your oxygen needs are heavy and you must travel...tanks work best.

Oxygen cylinder duration chart

Available at www.namdet.org

National Association of Medical Device Educators and Trainers

Cylinder Size	CD	ZD	E	F	HX	ZX	G	J	CD	ZD	E	F	HX	ZX	G	J	CD	ZD	E	F	HX	ZX	G	J
Contents (litres)	460	605	680	1,360	2,300	3,040	3,400	6,800	230	303	340	680	1,150	1,520	1,700	3,400	115	151	170	340	575	760	850	1,700
Contents	Full (100%)								Half Full (50%)								Low (approx. 25%)							
Flow Setting (Litres/min) 15	30m	40m	45m	1:31m	2:33m	3:22m	3:47m	7:33m	15m	20m	22m	45m	1:16m	1:41m	1:53m	3:47m	7m	10m	11m	22m	38m	50m	57m	1:53m
12	38m	50m	57m	1:53m	3:11m	4:13m	4:43m	9:27m	19m	25m	28m	57m	1:35m	2:06m	2:21m	4:43m	9m	12m	14m	28m	48m	1:03m	1:10m	2:21m
10	46m	60m	1:08m	2:16m	3:50m	5:04m	5:40m	11:20m	23m	30m	34m	1:08m	1:55m	2:32m	2:50m	5:40m	11m	15m	17m	34m	57m	1:16m	1:25m	2:50m
8	58m	1:15m	1:25m	2:50m	4:47m	6:20m	7:05m	14:10m	29m	37m	43m	1:25m	2:23m	3:10m	3:33m	7:05m	14m	19m	21m	43m	1:11m	1:35m	1:46m	3:33m
7	1:06m	1:26m	1:39m	3:14m	5:28m	7:14m	8:05m	16:11m	33m	43m	48m	1:36m	2:44m	3:37m	4h	8:05m	16m	21m	24m	48m	1:22m	1:48m	2h	4h
6	1:16m	1:40m	1:53m	3:47m	6:23m	8:27m	9:27m	18:53m	38m	50m	57m	1:53m	3:11m	4:13m	4:43m	9:27m	19m	25m	28m	57m	1:35m	2:07m	2:32m	4:43m
5	1:32m	2h	2:16m	4:53m	7:40m	10:06m	11:20m	22:40m	46m	1h	1:08m	2:16m	3:50m	5h	5:40m	11:20m	23m	30m	34m	1:08m	1:55m	2:32m	2:50m	5:40m
4	1:55m	2:30m	2:50m	5:40m	9:35m	12:40m	14:10m	28:20m	57m	1:15m	1:25m	2:50m	4:47m	6:20m	7:05m	14:10m	28m	37m	43m	1:25m	2:23m	3:10m	3:33m	7:05m
3	2:33m	3:21m	3:46m	7:33m	12:46m	16:53m	18:53m	37:46m	1:16m	1:41m	1:53m	3:46m	6:23m	8:27m	9:27m	18:53m	38m	50m	57m	1:53m	3:11m	4:13m	4:43m	9:27m
2	3:50m	5h	5:40m	11:20m	19:09m	25:20m	28:20m	56:40m	1:55m	2:31m	2:50m	5:40m	9:35m	12:40m	14:10m	28:20m	57m	1:15m	1:25m	2:50m	4:47m	6:20m	7:05m	14:10m
1	7:40m	10:05m	11:20m	22:40m	38:20m	50:40m	56:40m	113:20m	3:50m	5h	5:40m	11:20m	19:10m	25:20m	28:20m	56:40m	1:55m	2:31m	2:50m	5:40m	9:35m	12:40m	14:10m	28:20m

Nominal Time left in cylinder (in hours and minutes)

Note: Cylinder times are based on nominal content of cylinders and the nominal flowrate settings. Nominal contents can vary by +/- 5%. Nominal Flowrates can vary by +/- 20% (+/- 30% for 1 lpm) Some times (minutes) may be rounded up and or down

RED = 30 minutes or less	Amber = 31 minutes to an hour	Green = An hour or more

Note, every effort has been made to verify the actual times for each size cylinder. If there are any discrepancies or errors please inform us at enquiries@namdet.org ©Copyright NAMDET January 2021

Be certain to become educated about safety when dealing with oxygen. This gas is highly flammable. Do not try to cook while on oxygen. Another factor is making sure you have access to your oxygen at all times. Many do not realize the coordination required when dependent on oxygen. Your every move needs to be carefully planned in advance. You will need backups.

With a sufficient oxygen hose, you can generally travel through most of your house. The maximum length is 50 feet. It's good to purchase a supply of supporting materials because hoses and cannulas must be changed regularly. The cannula tends to stiffen and shrink over time, restricting oxygen flow. Keep an eye on it and have backups. When you "graduate" to a 10L unit you must use a High Flow (HF) cannula.

Keep in mind that the hoses often become kinked and cut off the oxygen flow. Always check your hose for that, especially where it comes to your face. You often can miss a problem there, I did.

As your oxygen needs increase, you will likely also have to have concentrated oxygen in tanks available. Pure oxygen is supplied in the tanks which is a higher concentration than the oxygen concentrators. Concentrators provide about 90% oxygen while tanks give 100% oxygen. These can be useful on those occasions when you find yourself particularly out of breath. Raise it to a higher level than normal for a few minutes until you have recovered from being short-winded. Keep it close; it's on wheels. You never want to place any low oxygen strain on your heart or brain.

Another necessary component in the mix is a good Pulse Oximeter. You place this on your finger to measure oxygen concentration in your blood and heart rate. It is essential to keep it above 90%. When you feel short breath, measure your concentration. That may determine the need for tank oxygen to rapidly catch up. Keep your oximeter and oxygen near you at all times and check regularly.

Oxygen is now an important element in your life. Educate yourself about your needs and what is available that best serves those needs. Also, remember that after transplant the occasion may arise when you will need oxygen again for a short duration. Do not give your equipment away!

The Diagnosis

Patients facing a lung transplant are often shocked to get the diagnosis. It comes about through a variety of ways. Sometimes a patient suffers from breathing issues and seeks medical attention. These individuals expect to have some sort of pulmonary problem. Their stress comes with the actual diagnosis.

On too many instances regular doctors miss the underlying cause of breathing problems. If you are having difficulties, see a pulmonologist. Interstitial Lung Diseases are too often misdiagnosed. Any delay can cause future problems.

In some cases, like mine, it is a total surprise. I attended my regular cardiac appointment only to have the young doctor on a fellowship hear something odd through his stethoscope. He said: "I hear something." I responded: "I hope it's my heart." He called in his mentor who agreed that something was amiss. They suggested that I make an appointment with a pulmonologist…which I did.

That appointment, after CT scan, 6-minute walk, and pulmonary function tests resulted in an initial diagnosis of Idiopathic Pulmonary Fibrosis (IPF) and the doctor informed me that my life expectancy was three to five years, perhaps a little longer. This was a total shock.

When I arrived home, my wife and I hugged and cried together. Our life had taken a stark change. Having spent forty-seven years together in marriage and eight before that dating, we fully expected a longer life together in our "Golden Years." Apparently, it was not to be unless some miracle occurred.

This is devastating news for anyone. Feel free to cry, scream, and punch the wall! Hit bottom. It is necessary because a ball cannot bounce back up until it has hit bottom. We are no different. Allow yourself to crater, but don't stay there! Get off the floor, look in the mirror, and say: "Ok, I am fine, I am strong, and I will prevail over this! I've got this!" Only by doing so can you face what confronts you and prevail.

My niece Lindsay Ponstein worked for a different pulmonologist. When she learned of my diagnosis, she insisted that I meet her doctor. I made the appointment, had a CT scan, and met with Dr. Janine Parker. She was concerned. After reviewing the same data, she concluded that it might be Hypersensitivity Pneumonitis (HP). Which, if chronic, can result in a similar outcome... progressive pulmonary fibrosis.

After over a year under Dr. Parker's care, she decided that I should have an open lung biopsy in order to better comprehend what was happening. This was done, and the resulting pathology report was more confusing. There was no clear indication of any one problem. She decided that I should be seen by a research specialist. I am forever thankful for Dr. Parker's efforts.

She transferred my case to Tulane Medical under the care of Dr. Joseph Lasky. This is a wonderful and thorough doctor who has taken care of me for the past number of years. He told me that the results of the biopsy are generally the gold standard for diagnosis. In my case, not so much. It just made matters more uncertain. He, too, leaned towards Hypersensitivity Pneumonitis as one underlying cause.

I willingly became a "lab rat" whereby I took a variety of different treatments seeking to arrest the fibrosis. I continued with my three-month visits and testing. This included tests for acid reflux, a known cause of fibrosis. To slow the process, Dr. Lasky placed me on Mycophenolate, Prednisone, OFEV, Esbriet, and Tyvaso. Although it seems to have slowed the fibrosis, it continued to expand and my breathing ability degeneration continued.

After three years of seeing him, I kidded with him that if it helped his research, he could have my old lungs in exchange for some new ones. He looked at me and said, "That's where we are. Are you willing?"

My response was: "Do I have a choice?" His response was: "Not really, if you wish to get better." Decision made. Your doctor must make a "Referral" to a transplant hospital. He referred me to Baylor St. Luke's in Houston where I began the long and arduous process of pre-testing for transplant approval.

Some are fearful when the issue of transplant arises. That is understandable, until you consider the alternative... a slow death through asphyxiation. It then becomes a door to a longer and better life. Talk with post-transplant patients and learn the advantages. I was supposed to die in 2021. I am still alive and kicking in 2026, five years after a Single Lung Transplant (SLT).

DO IT!!!!!

Preparations for Transplant Assessment

Conditioning

This is your Super Bowl! Prepare for it! If you are not in your top physical condition, this means you may not qualify for a transplant. Your body weight must be below 30 BMI (Body Mass Index). Calculators are available online. Otherwise, you could be denied for being unfit.

Hospitals are financed through Medicare, Medicaid, and Private Insurance; transplant programs cannot exist without this financial base. If they lose this income, the program ends. These groups require a high success rate, at least 90% over a year. That is why they must be so selective about choosing candidates. Transplant failures end programs.

Transplant and recovery play hard on the body. If you are overweight, you have challenged your entire system. The Hospital cannot take a chance on someone who's not healthy. You become "High Risk" which is a difficult proposition if self-induced.

This entire experience with lung disease means you must exercise as much as you can to stay in shape. If you want a lung transplant…work for it! Exercise, walk, eat right, get proper rest, be prepared as if an athlete before the big game because this is your "Big Game"! I used a variety of YouTube workout videos to build my strength and free weights to build my upper body.

It is important to develop a routine. Few enjoy doing exercise, but in this instance, it is so very important. In fact, scheduled exercise will become a necessary component of your life from now on.

You should try to walk as much as circumstances allow. Walking is the best exercise, and you will need strong legs and heart during your recovery. Remember, while in the hospital your strength will diminish by about 10% a day. So, you must build reserve strength as best as possible. You will need it after surgery and during recovery. The stronger you are, the less time you will spend in the hospital. I did not need physical therapy because I prepared myself for the experience.

Your entire quality of life depends upon good conditioning. This is especially true when seeking a transplant. So, start early!

Referral

There are many hospitals that perform Lung transplants. Your pulmonologist likely has a preferred institution that they commonly use for their patients. Convenience and a strong success record play a strong role in the decision. Since every hospital does not perform transplants, there is a good chance you may have to travel out of state.

Therefore, the hospital you will be referred to may not be in your neighborhood. You need to be within an hour or at most two hours from the Transplant Hospital. When a lung arrives, it has a short period of viability. You must be near the facility before it arrives. That is why most patients move close to the hospital in advance.

This can create a financial burden because there are the costs of maintaining a household in a distant city. In our case it cost us $24,000 that we were out of town, just for housing and food over the eight months we were in Houston.

Making arrangements for living near the hospital and for the transplant process is essential. Be prepared, you may be required to stay for an extended period of time. In my case it was eight and a half months total. That was for arrival, listing, transplant, and recovery. Often just waiting for a lung can take that long. Your assigned social worker can help with finding affordable housing.

Before embarking on the transplant journey, several matters must be considered. Many have no relation to your medical condition.

Does your health insurance cover the necessary medical expenses? Most do NOT cover housing or personal expenses while out of town. You must find the means of paying for that yourself. Be certain your insurance covers all MEDICAL EXPENSES. You want to be certain that you are not saddled with high medical costs along the way. That can destroy a family. The transplant process can exceed $1,000,000. Post transplant visits and procedures can double that.

Do you have disability insurance or does the business you work for have it? Family Leave is often available. Some pay during the leave; others do not. Do they guarantee that you will have a job when you return? Hopefully, it also provides some income while you are away. You will be gone from home for several months to a year. You need to know about this.

You will need an attorney. You must draft a will, Declaration Concerning Life Sustaining Procedures; you might consider Power of Attorney, Living Will, etc. as well as planning a funeral. The last is alarming but necessary. You likely should have done that already. You might consider a death doula cohort to help with your planning.

It is a shame that so many legal documents must be drafted, but it is necessary. Those relating to end of life are essential for the hospital providing your care. Others are merely a matter of covering bases in the event all goes sideways. Things happen, and you may not be in the condition to contend with them. Having this done in advance will prevent your family from chaos if you pass or become incapacitated. Having someone to take charge that knows what you want can relieve a lot of stress.

Transportation can be a serious issue. In my case, I was on a 10L concentrator at rest and 25L when active. It was a six-hour drive to the hospital. How do I have enough oxygen for the trip? Fortunately for me, my dear friend had a large motor home. He put me in, connected the concentrator to the vehicle generator, and off we went. This is a very serious consideration. You will not be going to a transplant center unless you are significantly oxygen compromised. Plan for this!

If the hospital is not in your locale, the process will require you to leave your home on several occasions for tests, surgery, and recovery. This can take weeks initially and later months as you await a donor lung and recovery after. Once surgery takes place, your absence can be much longer. Many hospitals require at least six-month for local recovery.

Where do you live? Is it close to the hospital? Must you move for a period of time? How do you handle responsibilities back at home while you are absent? What will be the cost and how will you cover it? What support do you have? What about transportation and other essentials, especially if your condition deteriorates? You cannot drive for months after surgery. These are important issues that must be considered in advance of your first appointment with the Transplant Pulmonologist.

You must have some savings to cover expenses. This is an essential component of your transplant review. Since insurance too often does not cover housing, that becomes a personal expense. Renting an apartment for many months on top of maintaining your existing home can become a serious financial burden. Be prepared.

Household bills have to be addressed. Your family must budget for those additional living expenses. Who cuts the lawn? Who maintains the house inside and out? Cars? Garden? All these issues must be considered as well as the cost. Which means sitting down and carefully developing a budget to cover both households.

Today some issues are not so difficult. You can have your bills either withdrawn from your account, or you can have them emailed and pay them through a bank bill pay. However, that requires setting up this process in advance to cover all bills. Make these arrangements ahead of time.

If you have a pet, this can create a whole host of other issues. Housing and caring for pets must be addressed as well. It is not easy to have a friend or relative play host to your pet for months on end. This is especially the case if they are older or if the pet has medical issues. Also, pets and certain plants and flowers cannot be in your environment post-transplant. The emotional side of this can be daunting, but necessary to solve.

The mail! What to do about your mail. One would think this would be easy and at an earlier time it would be. However, the postal service is not what it was. Getting mail forwarded to a second location can be problematic. If the mail is late or does not arrive, bills can fall behind. Important information may get lost. Also, since you may be having to change housing while out of town (later about that) the mail process will have to be done a second time, which creates a greater opportunity for error.

In our case, family members, Charlie and Claudette Ponstein, living next door picked up the mail daily at the house, reviewed it, and then put all the mail into an envelope, and mailed it to us. This prevented any mishaps. It also allowed us to return home when the opportunity arose without having to make further arrangements with the post office about our mail. Our family members also cared for our home while we were gone… one cannot fully express the thankfulness we have for them.

Housing is a major issue. If your hospital is not within two hours of your home, you may have to relocate for about a year. Perhaps less, but do not count on getting home early. Plan for a longer time and be thrilled if it is less. Maintaining two households on a limited budget can be difficult.

This is especially difficult for working families and those with children. Many lack any kind of savings, this makes financing living out of town daunting. Who will care for the children while their parent is out of town? Do you bring them with you, after all, you may be gone for nearly a year? You must make arrangements to care for your children, especially the young children, because some transplant housing will not allow children under 10 to stay unless they are patients themselves. The finances, education, emotions, and stress involved in this decision impacts your health. Be careful. There is help if you contact the hospital social worker. They are there for you.

Thankfully, there are facilities near most transplant hospitals that provide affordable housing. You will have to do some research. The transplant hospital's social worker often can help with this as well. They will provide a list. But it is up to you to research and find what suits you best.

In Houston we discovered a wonderful facility called Nora's Home. This establishment provides very affordable housing near the entire Houston medical complex. It was founded by two doctors who lost their young child and donated her organs to other children. During the process they discovered the problem with patient housing, so they established a foundation and constructed Nora's Home named after their much-loved child.

Nora's Home has thirty-two suites each with two queen beds and a full handicap accommodating bathroom. Occupants are required to provide their own food, but on occasions volunteers bring in wonderful meals as a treat. Large kitchens, a media room, exercise room, two dining rooms, library, computer room, and an outside patio further add to the ambiance of the facility. Nora's Home comes at an affordable cost based upon income. For some, it comes at no cost. This can relieve a lot of stress and makes your decision far less of a financial burden.

What matters most is the friendly staff and the communication one develops with other transplant patients. This is valuable because one meets people needing a transplant and those who have already completed the process. Do not be shy... meet and greet. Make friends here. Some have gone through what you are about to experience. You will learn so much from them.

The importance of this cannot be overstated. If you take the time, you will make life-long friends. We did! You will also develop a valuable resource for information. What other patients provide cannot be learned from books or seminars. Their stories provide guideposts.

There are other accommodations similar to Nora's Home near medical centers throughout the country. Take the time to research each for its proximity to your hospital and if it can accommodate your needs. Many only allow a ninety-day stay. That means that back-up plans must be established in the event of a longer recovery. Making reservations in advance is vital.

There may be apartments available. These can be convenient and within your budget if you must plan to relocate to another facility. If so, consider a two-bedroom so you can have visitors stay. There are costs involved that you must cover. Figure at least $3,500 per month at a minimum to cover food, hospital parking, and housing. That means that basic housing and food might cost about $36,000 for a year, perhaps more. So be prepared for this expense.

Many patients turn to various fund-raising efforts to help cover the expenses. The hospital social worker can help with this by providing information. Prepare for this in advance because this is what the transplant team needs to know... can you afford this expense? It serves no purpose to embark upon this journey if you lack the needed funding. Sadly, economics can come into play but be sure to check with the hospital social worker about assistance.

Parking is an expense during the wait for surgery, surgery, recovery and medical visits. At $17 per day for valet parking and $12 for daily parking it can easily come to $362 to $510 per month. But remember, you will only be in the hospital for a limited time, unless there are unforeseen complications. Therefore, you should consider a monthly pass initially to save money. That is about $80 a month. Parking passes are only issued after transplant. Some places like Nora's Home provide free shuttles to the hospital. Check on that too.

Housing can be cheap or sometimes even free if you take the time to research. The assigned hospital social worker will be of benefit in this regard. Some places do have time limits on staying. 90 days appears to be the norm.

Therefore, you will have to search for a second or third housing location while there. Unless you rent an apartment. We used three.

However, apartments can have problems. Some apartment complexes are very noisy. Neighbors above and beside can be a problem. You will need your rest. Also, you must consider safety. Some apartment neighborhoods have issues with crime and vandalism, especially regarding cars. Be mindful of that when planning and ask locals about the situation..

As for the home front, one never knows how long you will be gone. It is not just one journey. The first is relatively short. Meeting the Transplant Pulmonologist for a personal evaluation and conversation about the process. Following that, other meetings will take place with the entire Transplant Team, then several returns may be necessary to have medical tests performed. That can take a week or longer. In my case, the total process took nearly five months to complete all the testing. There were delays in getting the necessary appointments for tests arranged. (I will get into the tests later). Make sure you and your caregivers are present at every meeting. They need to see that you have a dependable support system. Also, take notes or ask to record these doctor meetings. You are given a great deal of information and the emotional state you are in can determine what you remember and hear.

Planning each trip takes time and careful consideration. What clothes to bring, what food to bring (if any), what does the housing provide, what stores deliver groceries, and sites like Amazon are a comfort. If you are on oxygen how will the tanks be delivered? A portable concentrator (Inogen) with back-up batteries might suffice. If you have higher needs, you may have to transport your 5L or 10L constant flow generator. You may even need to bring tanks as a back-up. If you bring tanks you have to find a local company that can provide refills.

There are organizations like Angle Flights that will fly you to appointments for free. Look them up on the internet and check them out. Sometimes the drive can be quite long. Angel Flights require a 10-day notice. As for commercial flying, you must check because most airlines will not allow oxygen tanks and your ability to breath at altitude may be compromised. If you want to bring a portable oxygen concentrator, that must be cleared with the airline in advance.

When placed on the transplant list you may be gone for many months. First the wait for a lung, then the surgery, and finally the recovery which comes with a period of post-transplant evaluation. Unless you live close to the hospital, you will be expected to stay near your hospital for several months, sometimes as long as a year. That is why the move may be necessary. Regular tests and check-ups are needed. You must be close by in the event of a sudden turn of events.

Why so long away? Again, hospitals are graded on success rates. If a hospital has issues with patient mortality Medicare and Insurance Companies will refuse coverage. That kills a program. They are judged on the first-year survival rate. Thus, they want you close by in the event of any complication so they can address it within that first year. That is also why they may limit taking on high risk patients, which is sad because an algorithm determines your life.

This is MAJOR surgery, make no mistake about that! There are differences in outcomes for Single Lung Transplant and Double Lung Transplant. The recovery time is less for single lung transplant. However, it seems that life expectancy for a double lung is better. Read up on this.

The risks are as high as are the rewards. Lung transplants have the highest percentage of rejections, and this can come about quickly. Even a minor lung infection like a cold, flu, or bronchitis can evolve into something very serious in the transplant world. Therefore, you must be near the hospital. Your life depends upon it! That's why you will be living close until the doctors feel comfortable that you have passed the danger stage... six months to a year depending on your experiences.

You must also obey EVERY protocol. Never change a med or add a med without contacting your coordinator. If you feel ill in any way, contact your coordinator. You made an agreement with them at the onset. Live up to it!

If you have all variables on the home front covered, that will relieve unneeded stress during the transplant process. You must devote 100% of your energy to recovery. You should not be anxious or distracted by outside matters. It is a lot to do, but you must do it.

Lastly, take the time to gather all of the medical information available on your case and place it in an easily accessible format. I created a table of contents with dates and placed this in a ring binder, so the pulmonologist had an easy time with it. You should have this for the first meeting. It should include medical procedures you have experienced, medication list, your doctors, and test results. Along with financial information, insurance, and a list of people who can support you. This last one is critical because you will need help.

In fact, two members of your support group should accompany you to all meetings. They must know what is going on, and it sends a clear message about commitment to the transplant team.

Perhaps most important is convincing the Pulmonology Team that you have the needed support, determination, strength of character, dedication, and financial resources to succeed. Firmly inform the transplant team that you WANT TO LIVE and will do everything asked to achieve that end. This especially means following ALL orders.

But be prepared to have to take family leave, sick leave, or disability. Doctors want total dedication to your health, no distractions.

Still working and being an active member of your community can be of benefit as well. They have to get to know you as a person. They must see your vitality. You must put your best foot forward. At 73 I was still teaching at my college full time online. Sell Yourself!!

The Testing Process

You will be called and informed of the date for your first appointment. That is why it is essential that you have all your homework completed. Included in these are arrangements for your housing and other needs. In my case, when I went to Houston Methodist I expected a short introductory visit with the pulmonologist. He placed me in the hospital and was there until transplant and recovery… about a month. Be prepared for the unexpected!

Your first visit will likely be for just a few days. You will meet your pulmonary Transplant team for an interview. Then tests will be scheduled, and you will return for those. As they schedule more tests, you will have to return to stay a week or more. Be prepared! I spent three months going to Houston from New Orleans for testing before being refused the transplant.

The odyssey began for us with a trip to St. Luke's to meet the Pulmonary Transplant Pulmonologist. If you require oxygen beyond a simple portable concentrator, be certain to contact the hospital in advance for the availability of a wheelchair and oxygen. It is generally accessible upon request and available at the valet parking.

You will meet the pulmonologist one-on-one but be certain to bring your support persons (two) with you. More on that later. But their role is so important that the transplant team must know who they are and meet them.

The doctor proved to be a very engaging gentleman who reviewed the medical records I had advanced. The doctor explained the entire process to me and educated me about the fact that acceptance into the program is not a certainty that I will receive a transplant. An entire medical review board makes the final decision. He asked pertinent questions, then listened to me. It was a good interview. A follow-up appointment was scheduled.

These medical tests were conducted during a follow-up visit some weeks later:

1. DLCO (Single Breath Diffusion):
    a. *Carbon monoxide diffusing capacity (Dlco) probably is the least understood pulmonary function test (PFT) in clinical practice worldwide, even among experienced pulmonologists. Every clinician knows that Dlco measures the quantity of carbon dioxide (CO) transferred per minute from alveolar gas to red blood cells (specifically hemoglobin) in pulmonary capillaries, and that this value, expressed as mL/min/mm Hg, represents mL of CO transferred per minute for each mm Hg of pressure difference across the total available functioning lung gas exchange surface.*[1]
2. Lung volume without Bronchodilator:
    a. *Bronchodilator drugs improve lung emptying, and this leads to variable increases in forced expiratory volume in 1 s (FEV$_1$), mainly by reducing lung volume rather than changing the FEV$_1$/forced vital capacity (FVC) ratio 5.*
3. CT test without IV contrast:
    a. *Computed tomography (CT scan or CAT scan) is a noninvasive diagnostic imaging procedure that uses a combination of X-rays and computer technology to produce horizontal, or axial, images (often called slices) of the body. A CT scan shows detailed*

images of any part of the body, including the bones, muscles, fat, organs, and blood vessels. CT scans are more detailed than standard X-rays.

4. Spirometry:

    a. Spirometry assesses the integrated mechanical function of the lung, chest wall, respiratory muscles, and airways by measuring the total volume of air exhaled from a full lung (total lung capacity [TLC]) to maximal expiration (residual volume [RV]). This volume, the forced vital capacity (FVC) and the forced expiratory volume in the first second of the forceful exhalation (FEV$_1$), should be repeatable to within 0.15 L.

5. *6-minute walk:*

    a. The 6 Minute Walk Test is a sub-maximal exercise test used to assess aerobic capacity and endurance. The distance covered over a time of 6 minutes is used as the outcome by which to compare changes in performance capacity.

Spirometry

The spirometry test is a comprehensive evaluation of your ability to breathe. This is the most important test you will likely be taking. Doctors evaluate your condition before transplant and your progress after transplant based on these results.

There are a lot of components to this test. This is not a complete list, but this breakdown should help you understand just what is being measured. Granted, a lot of these components are almost beyond comprehension for the untutored mind. But at least you will have some idea about what they are measuring.

1. FEV1 Pre - A derived value of FEV1% is FEV1% predicted, which is defined as FEV1% of the patient divided by the average FEV1% in the population for any person of similar age, sex, and body composition. (only you doctor will understand this)

2. FEV1 Predicted- Forced expiratory volume in one second, or the volume of breath exhaled with effort in one second. For the major components of spirometry (forced expiratory volume in 1 s (FEV_1), forced vital capacity (FVC) and FEV_1/FVC), the lower limit of normal (LLN), representing the lower 5% of test results from a normal population, differentiates a normal from an abnormal value.

3. FVC - *Forced vital capacity (FVC)* is the amount of air that can be forcibly exhaled from your lungs after taking the deepest breath possible. The full amount of air that can be exhaled with effort in a complete breath.

4. FEV1/FVC% - In general, your predicted percentages for FVC and FEV1 should be **above 80%** and your FEV1/FVC Ratio percentage should be above 70% to be considered normal. However, the information provided in these spirometry results can be used in many additional ways.

5. FEF 25-75% - Among the various measurements collected during conventional spirometry, forced expiratory flow at 25% and 75% of the pulmonary volume (FEF_{25-75}) measures the average flow rates of medium-to-small airways during the forced vital capacity (FVC) segment to testing and presents the status of those airways in patients.

6. PEF - The measurement is also called the peak expiratory flow rate (PEFR) or the peak expiratory flow (PEF). Peak flow measurement is mostly done by people who have asthma. Peak flow measurement can show the amount and rate of air that can be forcefully breathed out of the lungs.

There are several additional measurements that are difficult to explain to the uneducated in pulmonology. The above are the common terms you should understand when reading your test results. If you ask, your pulmonologist will take the time to explain the terms to you. It is important that you understand them well enough to be able to read the results and comprehend the condition of your lungs. Are they getting better, getting worse, or stable?

The purpose for all these tests is to give each institution its own data on your pulmonary condition. Some hospitals may require you to repeat these two tests nearly every time you come for an appointment.

After these tests we returned home and waited for a call providing us with a schedule for our next visit. Most hospitals have an online system called MyChart. Be certain to access that site daily. Open an account on your phone and computer, then look at it perhaps several times a day. Important information suddenly appears there, and they expect you to read it. This is critical to do!

We returned to Houston weeks later for additional tests and a meeting with the pulmonology team. This included a pulmonologist, the surgeon, a social worker, a financial person to discuss insurance, and personal ability to meet necessary expenses, a physical therapist who examined my strength, dietician, and pharmacist. Finally, I was introduced to a person who would become my "go to person." This was my contact with the hospital and team, my Coordinator. She was amazing. One key thing to remember is that the entire team wants you to succeed. They are there for you even if eventually you do not make the cut for a lung.

The delay in my second visit was attributable to the need to coordinate the multitude of tests in different buildings. I was on oxygen and moved from place to place by wheelchair. That had to be considered. Thanksgiving holiday did not help with the delay. No one to blame, just circumstances.

This second visit was the most critical. Be prepared! You will run a gauntlet of tests and physical exams. The purpose here is to discover any underlying health problem that might prevent you from being transplanted. Every organ is tested either by CT scan, x-ray, fluoroscope, echogram, or ultrasound just to begin with. Heart catheterizations were also performed. A weak heart can be a disqualifier.

Additionally, they must create a medical profile about you so, should you be accepted into the program, they will possess the necessary information for a perfect match with a donor.

The return required a seven-day stay, two for travel and five for testing. Many tests were conducted. Blood tests were first on the agenda. The Phlebotomist took twenty-three vials of blood at that time. They tested for over 70 different things. The remaining tests were clinical exams. The following provides information about the purpose of the tests:

Day one:

1. HL Carotid doppler Bilateral

   Carotid (kuh-ROT-id) ultrasound is a safe, noninvasive, painless procedure that uses sound waves to examine the blood flow through the carotid arteries. It also evaluates the thickness of the carotid artery wall and checks for clots.

2. HL Venous legs bilateral

   This test uses ultrasound to look at the blood flow in the large arteries and veins in the arms or legs.

3. 6-minute walk

   The 6 Minute Walk Test is a sub-maximal exercise test used to assess aerobic capacity and endurance. The distance covered over a time of 6 minutes is used as the outcome by which to compare changes in performance capacity.

4. Spirometry

   Spirometry is used to establish baseline lung function, evaluate dyspnea, detect pulmonary disease, monitor effects of therapies used to treat respiratory disease, evaluate respiratory impairment or disability, evaluate your operative risk, and perform needed surveillance for occupational-related lung disease. It may also be used in research and clinical trials and epidemiological surveys.

5. Blood Gas Arterial

   Blood gas analysis is a commonly used diagnostic tool to evaluate the partial pressures of gas in blood and determine acid-base content. Understanding and use of blood gas analysis enables medical providers to interpret respiratory, circulatory, and metabolic disorders.

Day two:

1. ABO grouping

   There are 4 main blood groups (types of blood) – A, B, AB and O. Your blood group is determined by the genes you inherit from your parents. Each group can be either RhD positive or RhD negative, which means in total there are 8 blood groups.

2. Sputum Culture + gram stain

   A sputum Gram stain is a laboratory test used to detect bacteria in a sputum sample. Sputum is the material that comes up from your air passages when you cough very deeply.

3. Histoplasma antigen, Urine

   Histoplasma antigen is detected using an enzyme immunoassay that detects Histoplasma galactomannan in urine. Reference value is a negative result which is consistent with the absence of infection. The presence of Histoplasma antigen in urine is indicative of current or recent infection with Histoplasma capsulatum.

4. HLA CII

   When the genetic marker HLA-DR4, a human leukocyte antigen that is a genetic anomaly, is found in white blood cells, there is a risk for developing RA.

The marker function is to distinguish one's own cells from foreign invaders. [2]. If HLA-DR4 cannot differentiate between the two, it may attack self-cells.

5. HLA CI

Results indicate how many antigens match and how many antigen mismatches are present. "0 mismatches" indicates a high probability that the organ or tissue will not be rejected by the recipient. The absence of recipient HLA antibodies to the donor HLA antigens is very important.

6. Urinalysis

Urinalysis is the physical, chemical, and microscopic examination of urine. It involves a number of tests to detect and measure various compounds that pass through the urine.

7. Hepatitis Quant RNA PCR

The viral load of hepatitis C refers to the amount of virus present in the bloodstream. The quantitative HCV RNA tests measure the amount of hepatitis C virus in the blood. The result will be an exact number, such as "1,215,422 IU/L."

8. AB Specificity Class I

The development of sensitive methods for alloantibody detection has been a significant advance in determining clinical transplantation. However, the complexity of the data from solid phase and crossmatch assays has led to potential confusion about how to use the results for clinical decision making. The goal of this review is to provide a *practical guide for transplant physicians for the interpretation of antibody data to supplement consultation with local tissue typing experts.*

9. CBC/Auto Differential:

<u>Red blood cells</u>, *which carry oxygen from your lungs to the rest of your body.*

☐ *<u>White blood cells</u>, which fight infections and other diseases. There are five major types of white blood cells. A CBC test measures the total number of white cells in your blood. A different test called a CBC with differential measures the number of each type of these white blood cells.*

☐ *<u>Platelets</u>, which stop bleeding by helping your blood to clot.*

☐ *<u>Hemoglobin</u>, a protein in red blood cells that carries oxygen from your lungs to the rest of your body.*

☐ *<u>Hematocrit</u>, a measurement of how much of your blood is made up of red blood cells.*

☐ *<u>Mean corpuscular volume (MCV)</u>, a measure of the average size of your red blood cells.*

10. Sjogren's Antibodies.

This test looks for two types of auto antibodies, SS-A and SS-B, which are commonly associated with Sjogren's Syndrome. Sjogren's is an autoimmune disease, a disorder in which a person's immune system turns against the body's own cells.

11. Antiscleroderma-70 Antibodies:

Scl-70 antibodies alone are detected in about 20 percent of SSc patients and are associated with the diffuse form of the disease, which may include specific organ involvement and chance of a poor prognosis. Scl-70 antibodies have also been reported in a varying percentage of patients with systemic lupus erythematosus (SLE).

12. Rheumatoid Factor Screen

A rheumatoid factor test measures the amount of rheumatoid factor in your blood. Rheumatoid factors are proteins produced by your immune system that can attack healthy tissue in your body. High levels of rheumatoid factor in the blood are most often associated with autoimmune diseases, such as rheumatoid arthritis and Sjogren's syndrome. But rheumatoid factor may be detected in some healthy people, and people with autoimmune diseases sometimes have normal levels of rheumatoid factor.

13. J0-1 Antibodies:

It is widely believed that patients bearing auto-antibodies to histidyl tRNA synthetase (anti-Jo-1) very likely to have a connective tissue disease including myositis and Interstitial lung disease. The value of positive tests in low disease prevalence settings such as those *tested in routine care is unknown. We sought to determine the value of anti-Jo-1 auto-antibodies in routine practice.*

14. Anti-DNA:

> *The anti-dsDNA test helps diagnose the presence of lupus when you have lupus signs and symptoms and a positive ANA (antinuclear antibody) test.*

15. Compliment C4\ Body Fluid:

> *This test measures the amount of C4 proteins in your blood. These proteins are an important part of your complement system, an important part of your immune system that helps kill disease-causing bacteria and viruses.*

16. Compliment c3\ Body Fluid:

> *A C3 complement blood test gives your healthcare provider information about your immune system. It shows how parts of your immune system are responding to harmful substances. This test can help your healthcare provider diagnose autoimmune disorders (like lupus), as well as other conditions.*

17. Antineutrophil Cytoplasmic A:

> *Antineutrophilic cytoplasmic antibody (ANCA) associated vasculitides are a heterogeneous group of rare autoimmune conditions that cause an inflammation of blood vessels with*

various manifestations. This activity outlines the clinical evaluation and management of ANCA-associated vasculitides and highlights the role of an interprofessional team in managing patients with this condition.

18. Aldose:

Aldose reductase catalyzes the conversion from glucose to sorbitol in mammals, which is the main cause of diabetic complications, such as cataracts and neurological diseases (Nishimura et al., 1991). Aldose reductase inhibitors can effectively inhibit the abnormal increase in the sorbitol content of the organs of diabetic patients, which can be used as active ingredients in the prevention and treatment of diabetes complications.

19. Flo PRA Class II with reflex:

The development of sensitive methods for alloantibody detection has been a significant advance in clinical transplantation. However, the complexity of the data from solid phase and crossmatch assays has led to potential confusion about how to use the results for clinical decision making. The goal of this review is to provide a practical guide for transplant physicians for the interpretation of antibody data to supplement consultation with local tissue typing experts.

20. Flow PRA Class I with Reflex:

*PRA stands for **Panel Reactive Antibodies**. In order to determine whether or not a patient already has any specific HLA antibodies, a lab specialist will test a patient's blood (serum) against lymphocytes (white blood cells) obtained from a panel of about 100 blood donors.*

21. Vitamin D 25 Hydroxy:

Doctors use the 25-hydroxy vitamin D test to monitor your vitamin D levels. Low levels can mean you need to spend more time outdoors or adjust your diet.

22. Varicella Zoster IGG:

Determination of immune status of individuals to the varicella-zoster virus (VZV). Documentation of previous infection with VZV in an individual without a previous record of immunization to VZV

23. TSH RFX Free T4:

Normal thyroid-stimulating hormone (TSH) levels generally fall between 0.4 and 4.0 milliunits per liter (mU/L). TSH levels higher than 4.5 mU/L usually indicate an underactive thyroid (hypothyroidism), and low TSH levels—below 0.4 mU/L—indicate an overactive thyroid (hyperthyroidism).

24. Toxoplasma Gond II Ab igG.:

A positive Toxoplasma IgG result is indicative of current or past infection with Toxoplasma gondii. A single positive Toxoplasma IgG result should not be used to diagnose

recent   infection.   Equivocal
Toxoplasma IgG results may be due
to very low levels of circulating IgG
during the acute stage of infection.

25. T Spot TB:

TB test is a blood test for TB
screening performed in one visit,
using one blood collection tube. The
T-SPOT.TB test is an in vitro
diagnostic test.

26. Strongyloides Antibody IGG:

It *is a parasitic disease caused by*
nematodes, or roundworms, in the
genus Strongyloides. The parasites
enter the body through exposed skin,
such as bare feet. Strongyloides is
most common in tropical or
subtropical climates.

27. Rubeola Ab IIgG:

Testing for suspected measles
infection should include rubeola *IgM*
and IgG   antibodies. *Positive*
IgG *with negative IgM results indicate*
immunity to infection.

28. RPR RFX QN/confirm TP.:

29. It *is a simple blood test that checks for*
unique syphilis antibodies. The RPR test
can be inconclusive on its own.

30. Rubella Ab IgG:

Rubella IgG antibody *can be formed*
following rubella *infection or after*
rubella *vaccination. A reactive result*
is consistent with immune status ...

31. Prostate- Specific AG\ Serum:

Elevated prostate-specific antigen (PSA) levels can be a sign of *prostate cancer*. It can also indicate noncancerous problems such as *prostate* ..

32. Dilute Prothrombin Time:

Prothrombin is a protein made by the liver. Prothrombin helps blood to clot. The "prothrombin time" (PT) is one way of measuring how long it takes blood to form a clot, and it is measured in seconds (such as 13.2 seconds). A normal PT indicates that a normal amount of blood-clotting protein is available.

33. Mumps IGG Antibody:

The presence of detectable IgG-class antibodies indicates prior exposure to the mumps virus through infection or immunization. Individuals testing positive are considered immune to mumps virus.

34. Lipid Panel w LDL/HDL Ratio:

Total cholesterol is a measurement of both good and bad cholesterol. LDL cholesterol moves cholesterol into your arteries. HDL cholesterol moves cholesterol out of your arteries. A high HDL cholesterol number lowers your risk for coronary heart disease. A high LDL cholesterol number raises your risk for coronary heart disease.

35. Immunoglobulin G (IGG):

This test checks the amount of certain <u>antibodies</u> called immunoglobulins in your body. Antibodies are <u>proteins</u> that your immune cells make to fight off bacteria, viruses, and other harmful invaders. The immunoglobulin test can show whether there's a problem with your <u>immune system</u>.

36. HIV-1 Antigen W/HIV 1&2 Antibodies:
All tests for HIV antibodies will look for HIV-1, which is more common than HIV-2 in the U.S. Combination tests have been developed to find HIV antibodies and HIV antigens called p24 antigens. The HIV antibody test advised by the CDC is the HIV-1/2 antigen/antibody combination immunoassay test.

37. Hepatitis Panel:
hepatitis panel *is a blood test that's used to find out if you have been infected with hepatitis A, hepatitis B, or hepatitis C virus.*

38. Hepatitis B Surface Antigen:

Detection of the Hepatitis B Surface Antigen in Patients with Occult Hepatitis B by Use of an Assay with Enhanced Sensitivity

39. Hepatitis B Surface Antibody:
For hepatitis B surface antibody (anti-HBs), a level less than 5 mIU is considered negative, while a level more than 12 mIU is considered protective. Any value between 5 and

12 mIU is indeterminate and should be repeated.

40. Hep B Core Antibody Total:

This *assay can be used as an aid in the diagnosis of individuals with acute or chronic* hepatitis *B virus* (HBV) *infection.*

41. Hepatitis Ab IgG:

A *positive result indicates the presence of HAV-specific IgG antibody from either vaccination or past exposure to hepatitis A virus.*

42. Hemoglobin A1C:

HbA1c is your average blood glucose (sugar) levels for the last two to three months. If you have diabetes, an ideal HbA1c level is 48mmol/mol (6.5%) or below. If you're at risk of developing type 2 diabetes, your target HbA1c level should be below 42mmol/mol (6%).

43. GSPD Quantitatively:

Glucose-6-phosphate dehydrogenase (G6PD) deficiency is an inherited disorder caused by a genetic defect in the red blood cell (RBC) enzyme ...

44. Epstein Barr Virus IGG.

Blood tests for Epstein-Barr *virus detect antibodies to EBV in the blood and help establish a diagnosis of EBV infection.* Epstein-Barr virus ...

45. Cytomegalovirus Ab IgG:

- A positive CMV IgG *and IgM when you have symptoms means it is likely that you have been exposed to* CMV

for the first time recently or a previous CMV *infection ...*

46. Cryptococcus Antigen\ Serum:

Early cryptococcal disease can be detected via circulating antigen in blood before fulminant meningitis develops, when early antifungal therapy improves survival.

47. Comprehensive Metabolic Panel:

— A comprehensive metabolic panel (CMP) is a test that measures 14 different substances in your blood. *It provides important information about ...*

48. Coccidioides ABS\ QN\ Did:

Coccidioides antibody test; Coccidioidomycosis blood test. Coccidioides complement fixation is a blood test that looks for substances (proteins) called antibodies, which are produced by the body in reaction to the fungus Coccidioides immitis. This fungus causes the dangerous disease coccidioidomycosis.

49. Type N Screen Automated:

Reliably type red blood cells antigens beyond traditional ABO Blood ... the NEO® made it possible for us to automate all type & screen samples on the NEO.

Day Three:

1. MN Lung Scan Quant Ventilation:

In the V/Q lung scan, an aerosol and injectable radioactive tracer are used to assess lung ventilation *(V) and perfusion (Q) to identify V/Q mismatch areas.*

2. HL PV Arterial ABI Unilateral:

    What does a high ankle-brachial index mean? An ABI ratio higher than 1.4 could mean the blood vessels in your limbs are stiff because of advanced age or diabetes. Researchers have found that people with an ankle-brachial index higher than 1.4 had twice the risk of cardiovascular death.

3. ECHO W Contrast &n Doppler:

    An echocardiogram is a noninvasive (the skin is not pierced) procedure used to assess the heart's function and structures. During the procedure, a transducer (like a microphone) sends out sound waves at a frequency too high to be heard. When the transducer is placed on the chest at certain locations and angles, the sound waves move through the skin and other body tissues to the heart tissues, where the waves bounce or "echo" off of the heart structures. These sound waves are sent to a computer that can create moving images of the heart walls and valves.

4. XR Chest 2 views:

    Typically, two views of the chest are taken, one from the back and the other from the side of the body as the patient stands against the image recording plate.

5. XR Bone density Study:

A *bone mineral density (BMD) test can provide a snapshot of your bone health. The test can identify osteoporosis, determine your risk.*

6. XR Mandible 4 views:

If you have low bone mass that is not low enough to be diagnosed as osteoporosis, this is sometimes referred to as osteopenia. Low bone mass can be caused by many factors.

7. FL Esophagus:

An esophagram is a kind of X-ray that takes video images of your esophagus in action. It's also called a barium swallow test.

8. FL Sniff Test:

The fluoroscopic sniff test, also known as diaphragm fluoroscopy, is a quick and easy real time fluoroscopic assessment of diaphragmatic ...

Day Four:

1. Cardiac Cath Report:

The usual arterial access route is via the radial or femoral artery. The diagnostic angiography report comments on each main epicardial artery in turn, starting with the left system. The left main stem (LMS) bifurcates into the left anterior descending artery (LAD) and left circumflex (LCx). Then the right coronary artery (RCA) is described (for common abbreviations see Box

1). On occasions branch vessels will also be described as a subset of their main epicardial vessel. The angiogram report may refer to either the LCx or the RCA as the 'dominant' vessel/territory, to indicate which of the two vessels gives rise to the posterior descending artery (PDA) branch.

2. Cardiac Cath Scan:

    A heart CT scan creates high-resolution images of your heart to assess for heart, valve, coronary artery, aorta and other diseases.

3. Creatinine Clearance @$ hr Urine:

    The measurement of accurate renal function is vital for the routine care of patients. Determining the renal function status can predict kidney disease progression and prevent toxic drug levels in the body.[2] The glomerular filtration rate (GFR) describes the flow rate of filtered fluid through the kidneys. The gold standard measurement of GFR involves the injection of inulin and its clearance by the kidneys.

4. Creatinine Serum:

    An increased level of creatinine *may be a sign of poor kidney function.* Serum creatinine *is reported as milligrams of* creatinine *to a deciliter ...*

5. ECG-12 Lead:

    As a non-invasive yet most valuable diagnostic tool, the 12-lead ECG records the heart's electrical activity as waveforms. When interpreted accurately, an ECG can detect and monitor a host of heart conditions - from arrhythmias to coronary heart disease to electrolyte imbalance.

6. POCT-ACT:

   To monitor treatment with heparin or other blood-thinning medications (anticoagulants) when undergoing heart bypass surgery, coronary angioplasty, or dialysis

7. Postassium- Stat Lab:

   A potassium *blood test measures the* potassium *levels in your blood. Too much or too little* potassium *may indicate a serious medical problem.*

8. Blood Gas Arterial:

   Arterial blood gas (ABG) analysis is an essential part of diagnosing and managing a patient's oxygenation status and acid–base balance. The usefulness of this diagnostic tool is dependent on being able to correctly interpret the results.

9. *Poct*-Glucose Meter:

   POC testing is a widely used tool to enable immediate determination of *glucose* levels in hospitalized patients and facilitate rapid treatment ...

10. ECG- Lead:

    Electrocardiograph is an Instrument used to record electrical activity of the heart, non-invasively, which reflects contraction and relaxation of Cardiac muscles in a Cardiac cycle.

11. Lipid Panel W Ldl/HDl Ratio:

Blood screening tests give you important information that can detect cardiovascular issues which may require treatment in the form of medication or lifestyle modification. Your results could also indicate that further testing is needed for a condition such as heart failure or stroke.

12. CBCw/Auto Differential:

A differential blood count is a blood test to check your white blood cell levels, which can indicate the presence of infection, disease, or an allergic reaction. Your doctor might order it as part of routine testing or to check for infections and other problems.

13. Blood Gas Venous:

Arterial blood gas analysis is used to measure the pH and the partial pressures of oxygen and carbon dioxide in arterial blood. The investigation is relatively easy to perform and yields information that can guide the management of acute and chronic illnesses. This information indicates a patient's acid-base balance, the effectiveness of their gas exchange and the state of their ventilatory control.

14. Lactic Acid Venous:

Lactic acid is produced in physiologically normal processes, and as a common finding in disease states. When increased production is comorbid with decreased clearance, the severity of the clinical course escalates. Importantly, the effects of severely elevated levels of lactic acid can have profound hemodynamic consequences and can lead to death.

15. PTT Activated:

A partial thromboplastin time (PTT) test measures the time it takes for a clot to form in a blood sample. It helps find bleeding.

16. Dilute Prothrombin Time:

Prothrombin time *(PT) is a blood test that measures the time it takes for the liquid portion (plasma) of your blood to clot.*

17. Phosphorus:

    a. Most commonly, a high level of phosphorus is related to a kidney disorder. It shows that your kidneys are having difficulty clearing phosphorus from your blood. A high level of phosphorus can also mean uncontrolled diabetes and other endocrine disorders.

Day Five:

1. Colonoscopy:

    a. Colonoscopy is a procedure in which a doctor uses a colonoscope or scope, to look inside your rectum and colon. Colonoscopy can show

irritated and swollen tissue, ulcers,
polyps, and cancer NIH external link.

All of the required tests for establishing suitability for transplant take time. Make sure you bring snacks and water with you. The next step was to meet with the transplant pulmonologist and surgeon for a last time before my case was to be presented to the Medical Review Board for a final decision. The composition of that body, which holds your life in their hands, is unknown to you.

They generally meet once a week in the morning to review the cases. The board will report one of three outcomes: "Yes", "No", "Deferred." The last one means that further information needs to be gathered. The first is a blessing, the second is depressing. But do not let it get you down. Many people are rejected on their first try. Other hospitals will take you, but you must apply. Be aggressive; your life depends upon it. It took two tries for me. I met a man who made nine attempts before success. Never give up! Never Yield!

In my case, the review board said "NO." From my understanding the surgeon held concerns about the strength of my heart which had stents and my age, me being 73 years old. Everything else was good. but who knows who or what was said in that meeting. There is no appeal to this decision.

We were told to wait for a phone call. If we heard a nurse's voice it's good news. If we heard from the pulmonologist, it was a rejection. The doctor called.

We were crushed. From October 2022 to the following March 2023, we invested resources, time, and energy in the process. Those five months took an emotional toll. I felt like my world had collapsed. It hadn't. Never get down. If one door closes, look for an open window, climb through the cellar. Never give up.

One must consider that each hospital has its own guidelines. The concern is about transplant failure. If a patient has complications or dies it goes into hospital's records. As mentioned earlier, if a hospital has too many failures both the government regulators in Medicare and insurance companies will discontinue support for the program. Some surgeons themselves are less inclined to take on any risky patients; it can hurt their reputation. While others believe that the process involves risks and are willing to take them. The larger the hospital transplant program, the more risks they will take.

After being notified of my rejection, the transplant pulmonologist was kind enough to transfer my medical records to two other hospitals and informed me that I should contact them. I immediately called the closest one, Houston Methodist, and an appointment was made.

Within a week of the call to Houston Methodist, I had an appointment scheduled. However, that appointment was six months away. My health situation was such that six months was not feasible. Do keep this in mind. I later contacted the hospital and asked if there was a cancellation I could take. I was informed that one was available within two weeks. I immediately took it. Remember, maintain contact with the transplant team and ask questions. This simple phone call may have saved my life. You need to advocate for yourself.

St. Luke's sent over all the medical records they had accumulated, and Houston Methodist reviewed them. I was notified that I needed two additional tests, but they could be performed at a local hospital. That was done and the test results sent to Houston Methodist.

Next came the meeting with their Transplant Pulmonologist at the second hospital. The process began again, only this time at a very fast pace.

Second Attempt
Houston Methodist

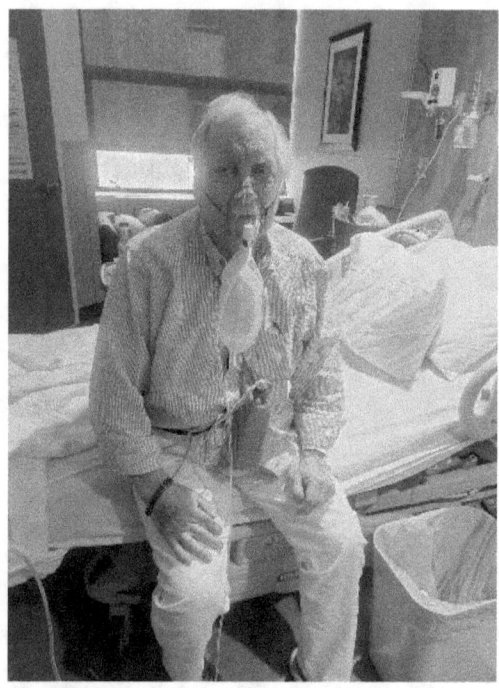

Arrival at Houston Methodist

We assumed the process would be the same at Houston Methodist. Meet the Pulmonologist, go home. Wait for an appointment with the Pulmonology team, go home. Schedule additional testing, go home. Then wait for a call informing me if I am listed.

As mentioned earlier, I was in desperate straits. Using 10L at rest and 25L with exertion. How to get to

Houston by car on impossible with 3L Inogen oxygen portable. This is a real problem for potential transplant patients. A dear friend saved my life. He put me and my 10L concentrator in his motor home and drove me there. Another friend traveled to Houston with eighteen cylinders of oxygen in a rented van.

A short visit was not to be. We left New Orleans, packed for only a 3 day stay, and came to Houston expecting a short visit. When we met the assigned pulmonologist, he spoke with us at length. After this visit he immediately arranged an appointment with a second Transplant Pulmonologist. This doctor spent the better part of an hour reviewing my medical records. He then had me admitted into the hospital as an in-patient for additional tests. I was placed in ICU.

They performed CT scans of the lungs, chest, and neck. Complete blood work (another 30 vials) full pulmonary function tests, additional CT scans, ultrasounds, sonograms, and x-rays. Within two weeks, everything needed was completed. This hospital moved at a fast pace.

Suddenly, one morning Dr. Koch entered my room and did a little dance. He informed me that the Medical Review Board approved my application for a lung transplant. I was so fortunate. It happened a mere fourteen days after entering ICU. The hospital then began the next step of entering all my information into the Organ Procurement & Transplant Network (OPTN). This is a national non-profit with a government contract that coordinates donors with patients and doctors.

Within a few days OPTN placed me on the transplant list once all insurance issues had been cleared. I was then given my CAS (Composite Allocation Score) which determines a number upon which priorities for lungs are determined. My score was 19.0975 which is about the normal range for transplant.

The Composite Allocate Score (CAS)

The Composite Allocate Score or CAS is the number assigned to each lung transplant patient that determines their priority on the transplant list. It is a complicated and moving number based upon a variety of variables. Rather than attempting to explain the process, it is presented here in the words of the Organ Procurement & Transplant Network (OPTN).

Every lung transplant candidate receives an individualized lung Composite Allocation Score (CAS). This score determines priority for receiving a lung transplant when donor lung(s) become available. The lung CAS is individual for each patient and each organ offer. The lung CAS point values represent each of the factors used to match organ offers with transplant candidates. The people who have the highest number of points for that organ offer will have the highest priority.

How is the lung CAS calculated?
The lung CAS uses objective medical information about your needs and medical condition. It also uses objective medical facts about the potential organ donors that may be a match for you. The score weighs the different factors used to make the match. This means each factor will get a certain number of potential points, which are then added together to make up a maximum score of 100 points. Some factors are more important in matching and will be worth more points within the overall score, while others get fewer points. Medical experts have carefully determined the weight for each factor

based on input from the donation and transplant community as well as detailed statistical information. Patients and the general public also provided input on the factors that they think are most important in determining how to place donor lung(s).

The lung CAS uses a framework called continuous distribution. Some of the goals of this framework are to:

- *Prioritize sickest candidates first to reduce waitlist deaths.*
- *Improve long term survival after transplant.*
- *Increase transplant opportunities for patients who are medically harder to match.*
- *Increase transplant opportunities for candidates with distinct characteristics like candidates under the age of 18 or prior living donors.*
- *Promote the efficient management of organ placement.*

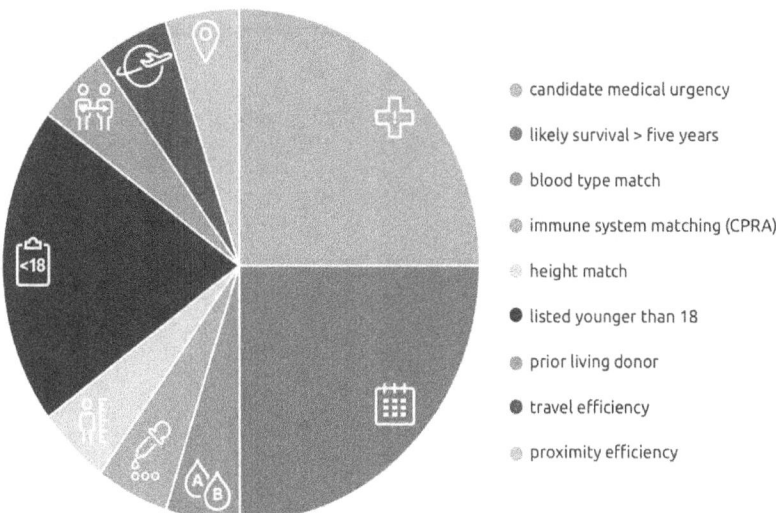

- candidate medical urgency
- likely survival > five years
- blood type match
- immune system matching (CPRA)
- height match
- listed younger than 18
- prior living donor
- travel efficiency
- proximity efficiency

Getting to this point proved to be a great achievement. It means that I have been accepted into the process for a lung transplant and have a CAS number. The higher the number the higher you are placed on the transplant list. The first sets of hurdles are over and the initial phase behind me. Then begins the wait for a donor lung to appear with my name on it. [1]

---

[1] https://www.cas.org/cas-data/cas-registry

The Wait

Waiting for a lung creates a whole new set of stresses. You must be available twenty-four hours per day and live within an hour of the hospital. That is why if you live remotely from the hospital, it is critical you find living arrangements close by. When the call comes, you and your caregiver must be ready to move... fast!

Donor organs become available randomly and have a short lifespan. Generally, availability is due to an accident or an overdose. The Transplant Team sends a surgeon over to retrieve the organ and assess its viability. Meanwhile, the chief Transplant Pulmonologist must review his CAS list and find the person most likely to benefit from the transplant then begin the process of arranging the surgery.

This waiting period can last for days, weeks, months, and even years. There is no advanced warning. Your telephone becomes your constant companion, and you cannot travel far from the hospital. You may think visiting distant friends and family for a short time is ok. It is not. What if you get the call while away?

Staying close sends a clear message about your willingness to abide by the rules. If they call and you are not available, you are passed up. I have no idea what the implications of that are for a future attempt, but it cannot be good.

This can be a strain on many levels, but a necessary one. If you get a transplant, you will have all the freedom you need to travel. So, invest the time. Non-compliance sends a clear message. Your transplant team is working very hard to save your life; your cooperation is essential. You just have to be patient and wait.

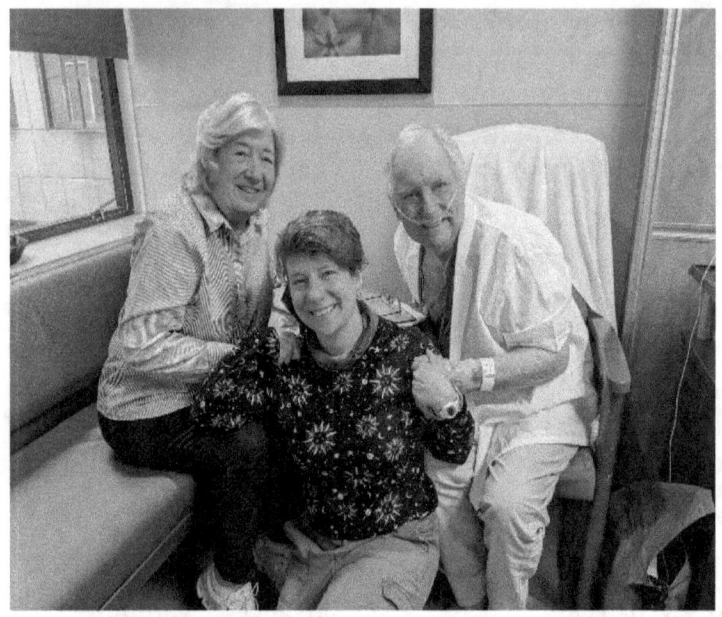

My Wife Margaret, Daughter Becca, and me...waiting

The Call

Be prepared... be very prepared! You and your caregivers must be packed and ready to move at a moment's notice. The call will come suddenly, and you must react immediately, but do not panic. It can happen at night or early in the morning. Bags must be packed in advance. Attitude tuned for the moment. Be ready!

My health had become critical. I began to realize that I would likely never see my home again, which is depressing. At rest I was using 10L liters of oxygen. When I walked, I used 25 liters.

Many do not survive to see a transplant. It's a strange mix. If you are critical and in ICU you move up the list. If you become too critical they may be forced to pass you over. At some point the fortunate ones will receive a call. It is sudden. Consider... overdoses and accidents occur in the early morning or weekends. As mentioned, these are the general sources for organ donations.

Once an organ becomes available, a surgeon from your transplant team will immediately travel to the donor's location to retrieve the organ. At this point he/she will examine it, test it, type it, and report the findings. Is it good for transplant or not? If good, the next person on the list will be contacted.

If your CAS number places you at the top, you will be immediately called and told to report to the hospital. Have a bag packed in advance with all the essentials you will need. This is no time for searching for items. Also have your support person readily available. They must accompany you to the hospital. Once there, you will be prepared for surgery.

74

You may or may not have an hour or two to prepare. You will learn from your Surgical team about a match by phone. It must be always charged and close by. Your transplant team will inform you as to where to report to the hospital. Your new journey has just begun. Just a short note... if you are a male, do yourself a favor... shave your upper body! They will be continuously putting sticky tabs on you to monitor your heart. They hurt when they come off.

When the lung arrives the surgeon will look over the donated lung to determine if he believes it is viable. If not, you experienced a dry run. Dry runs are not uncommon. Sadly, sometimes the lung loses viability in transport. If yes, surgery begins. The complexity depends upon whether it is a single lung transplant or a double lung transplant. Neither is a walk in the park. This is major surgery and complications often do occur.

In my case, after eighteen days in the hospital and a seriously deteriorating health situation at 1:14 AM a nurse walked into my room with two plastic bags full of empty vials, over thirty of them. I asked what for and she informed me that she needed blood samples because I had just been awarded a lung. I was set for a single lung transplant. This was a mere five (5) days after being listed. A miracle!

I called my wife and daughter and told them the news. Margaret immediately traveled to the hospital to be by my side. Becca had to fly in from California. My transplant coordinator met me in my room to fill out the necessary paperwork. I then called our dear friend in New Orleans who graciously flew in to be by my wife's side. It is important for support to have support at times like this.

Annie was a blessing. She stayed with Margaret in the waiting room while they conducted the surgery. It is a very tense situation.

The Surgery

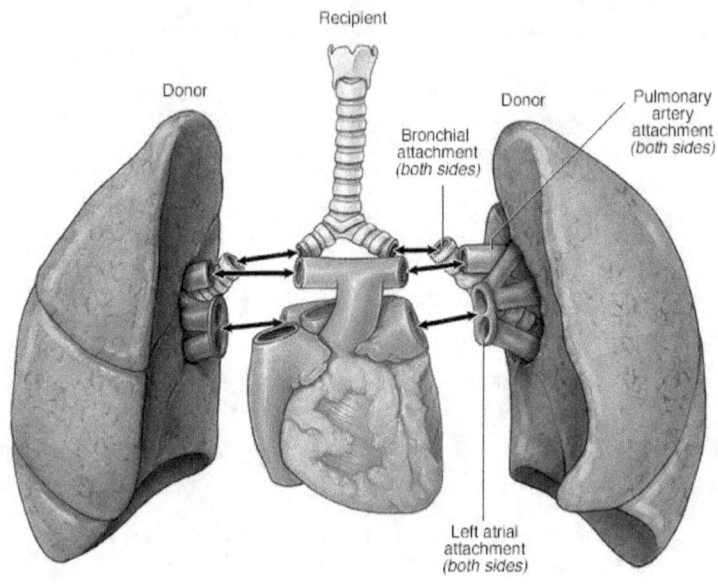

Recipient

Donor

Donor

Pulmonary
artery
attachment
(both sides)

Bronchial
attachment
(both sides)

Left atrial
attachment
(both sides)

Image Courtesy Mayo Clinic

You must remember that Lung Transplant surgery is a complicated and risky procedure. Although it will improve your quality of life, it comes with its own share of challenges.

The surgery cannot be performed if you have an active infection, recent personal history of cancer, serious diseases affecting other major organs, or indicate a hesitancy to make necessary changes post-surgery to protect the lung.

Also, you cannot have used illegal drugs...any illegal drugs.

When selecting the lung, doctors must consider many factors to make the match. That is why a multitude of tests are required. Blood, tissue type, size of lung, antibodies and lastly your health at time of surgery. If you are too ill, they cannot operate. If you have an infection, they cannot operate. You must stay isolated as much as possible while waiting.

Without getting into details, the surgeon must make an incision in your chest to remove the damaged lung. For a double transplant, this is across the chest to open the chest wall. However, they are beginning to use the single lung process for double lungs as well. For a single lung the surgeon opens the chest on the side of the damaged lung below the armpit. He enters between the ribs, expands them, deflates the lung, takes out the old lung and inserts the new one. In both cases the lung is inflated and examined. Following that the surgeon sutures connecting the blood vessels and Bronchial to the trachea. For a single lung there are only four attachments, eight for a double lung.

As mentioned earlier, I received a single lung. It happened fast! I was in the hospital bed reading at 1:14 pm when the door opened, and a nurse entered with a bag of empty blood vials. It was then that I was informed that I had a lung and would be in surgery later that morning.

A doctor flew out to get the lung while I was sent to pre-op for preparation at 5:40 AM 3rd floor Walter Tower. Dr. Suarez informed Margaret that the surgery could take 4-6 hours. Margaret visited me at 7:30 AM before I was rolled into surgery.

In the operating room at 7:58 AM. There was one hiccup. They had the jet to pick up the organ, but a pilot was not immediately available. Tension! Finally, one arrived and the trip to wherever took place. At 9:21AM final preparation began. 9:45AM lung is on the way and should arrive in 20-30 minutes. 12:15 PM surgery over… two hours and thirty minutes! A miracle. Bronchoscope performed then moved to CVICU by 2:00PM. Now it was just a matter of me waking up. This whole process was unusual. Eighteen days to list and five days to lung.

From surgery to recovery. Recovery was for a relatively short time. I was intubated and had a collection of tubes penetrating my chest wall. Heavily sedated. Felt no pain and do not recall being transferred to pulmonary ICU.

When I awoke, suddenly, the breath of life returned. I was still on oxygen but knew something was different. I could consider a future life with my family. Hope springs. I felt no fear about the surgery at all. It became my only hope to enjoy my family. Trust me, you will not fear this procedure…you will welcome it!

I knew my life had changed. No longer would I be tethered to 30 feet of plastic tubing. I would be able to do things I have not done in three years. I would be able to take a shower without oxygen, eat dinner without oxygen, leave the house and do almost everything I did before in life without oxygen. Yrs, there are limitations, but acceptable ones. Life is about compromises

Only those who have walked down this road can comprehend the stress of being forever breathless. People do take breathing for granted. When suffering from lung disease your every move must be orchestrated like a ballet. No longer!

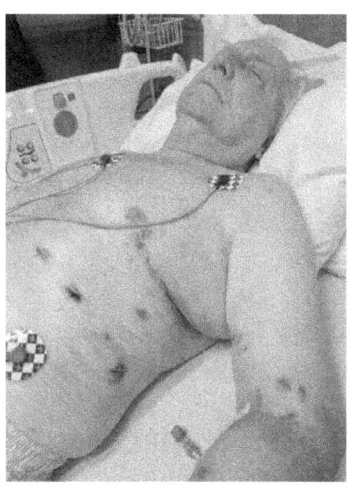

Single Lung Transplant… two Chest Tubes and one Incision

For obvious reasons I will have little else to say here. Once rolled into the operation theater, I looked around the room and observed the massive amount of equipment and the surgical staff. Most impressive. A nurse asked me if I had any metal objects on me, so I informed her that "*I have already removed my nipple rings!* (joke)". Always maintain a sense of good humor. The doctors, nurses, and staff experience a lot of stress during a major operation like this…do not add to it. Their sole intention is to make you well; necessarily some pain will be involved. Surprisingly, very little in my case, just at the incision site and chest tubes.

From surgery to the recovery room. Again, you will remember very little. You will be intubated so you cannot speak. DO NOT PANIC!!! To prepare for this, have some cue cards with words, phrases, or letters you can point to in order to communicate with loved ones and the medical team. A dry erase board will suffice too but know that your hands will be limited due to the needed restraints on your arms.

Also, writing is impossible. What I composed for my wife and staff was unreadable.

But remember, trying to write while under sedation can be humorous. When I saw what I tried to write to the nurse days later, it made no sense… scribble. Suggestion, don't even try. Relax and embrace the rest.

This recovery process is a very temporary situation in most cases. Again, much depends upon conditioning prior to surgery. If you are strong this will be short. If you have allowed yourself to become weakened, it could be longer. In other cases, a longer stay cannot be helped. Just a matter of post-surgery. Much is in your hands.

The Recovery

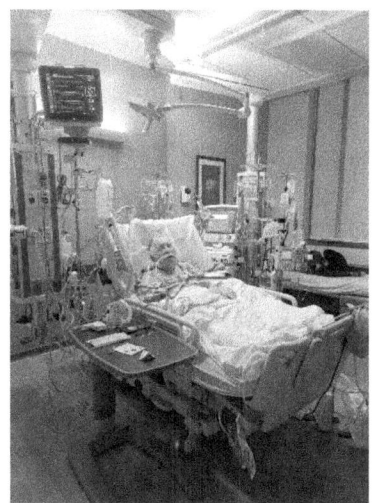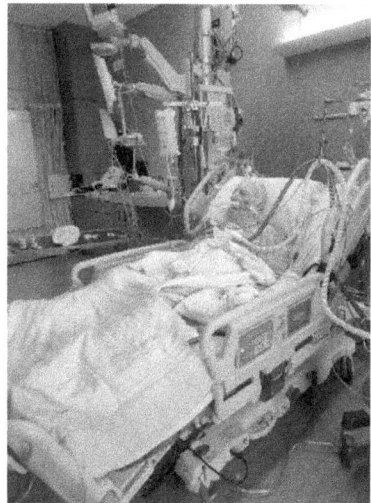

From Surgery to Recovery

Recovery takes as long as it takes. Some go through the process quickly, others do not. It depends upon a variety of variables mostly connected to your physical situation prior to surgery as well as your determination to recover after surgery.

When you get out you will resemble a humanoid. You will be on oxygen. Tubes will protrude from your body. You will be on a ventilator until such time as they are satisfied that you can breathe without one. You will have a feeding tube up your nose and into your stomach because they do not want you to aspirate while eating. You will have two chest tubes draining fluid post-surgery. You will have an IV for administering medicine, you will have a blood pressure cuff, and you will have a pulse oximeter attached to one of your fingers, and finally a heart monitor. These are all for observational purposes.

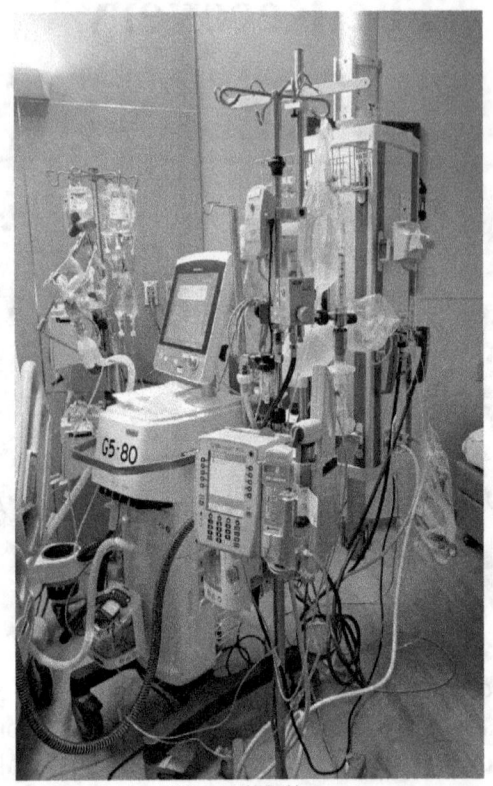
Your lifeline

This is what you will be connected to in recovery. There is an amazing amount of technology that monitors your condition and provides life support. It is impressive to watch the nurses manage this equipment.

Will you feel pain? Yes, but not what one would expect. You will likely only feel pain around the incision site when you move or cough. That is to be expected. This is especially the case when you walk, which you will do the very next day. The chest tubes move and generate local pain around the entry site when you move. Additionally, the muscles along the side of the incision move when walking which also hurts. They want you up and moving around ASAP to put your new lungs to work. The Physical Therapist will make you get up and walk. This hurts too because the chest tubes bounce and the muscles on your side by your incision will move.

DO NOT FEAR PAIN MEDS! What is most important is walking and movement. If pain inhibits you from walking, your recovery will be slower. I learned to take pain meds when walking. The nurses and doctors will not allow you to become addicted. Follow orders, walk, walk, walk and get better.

Over time they will gradually be removed except for pulse oximeter, blood pressure and IV which stay the whole while in recovery. The greatest pleasure is having the chest tube removed, but I must say, although this process does not hurt at all… it does feel weird!

Sleeping in an ICU can be an adventure. You are told to rest but rest you do not get. First, there is the ICU environment itself. Lights are constantly on; doctors and nurses are constantly on the move. This is one of the most active units in a hospital. Doctors and nurses are continually caring for patients, and this process is not overly quiet.

At Houston Methodist their helipad is located on the roof and the neighboring hospital's helipad is located outside my window. These are very active care facilities. All night long you hear engine noise. But do not be frustrated. Those are the sounds of hope. Patients or organs coming in to save lives.

The final issue pertains to your personal situation. You have just undergone very major surgical event. Complications are common. Therefore, you will be closely watched in the event of difficulty arising. This requires scrutiny of all systems. Make sure to communicate with your medical team. Let them know about any changes you are feeling. In my case, I started to hallucinate when I closed my eyes. Having mentioned it, the doctor simply changed my antifungal drug, and all was good. Talk about any issues you may have. Do not hesitate.

You will be immediately placed on 1000 mg Prednisone; your fingers will be pricked for glucose tests every hour for a period of time; then later every four hours. Your blood pressure cuff will inflate every thirty minutes. Multiple injections of various chemicals including immunosuppressives will be administered through your neck port. Heparin to prevent blood clots will become a part of your nightly regimen… a painless shot in the stomach. Insulin will likely be administered through a slight pinch of a shot in your upper arm. This is to control Hyper Glycemia from the prednisone. X-rays to check for your lungs condition, bronchoscopes to examine the interior of your lungs for complications, echograms to examine your liver and kidneys, the list goes on. You will also still be on oxygen. Expect that for a period of time until the new lung adjusts. Very little uninterrupted sleep. But all this is essential to secure your transplant and your life.

You will be up and walking on the very next day. It is essential to be sitting up and walking to exercise your new lungs. GET OUT OF BED!!! Sit up in the recliner for as long as you can. That is the only means of conditioning them. The goal is to become totally independent of oxygen.

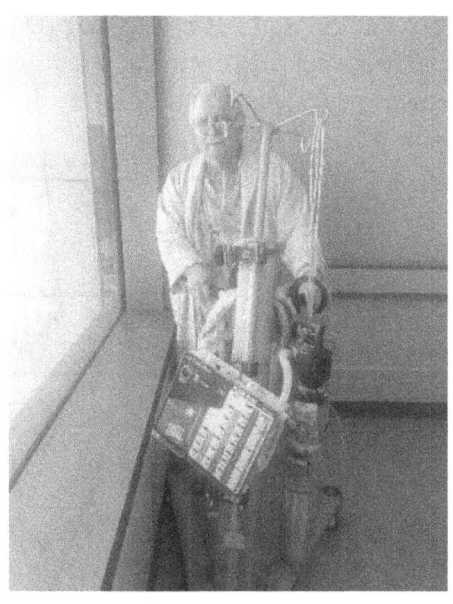

Walking One week after surgery

While in CVICU (Cardio/Vascular Intensive Care Unit) your feeding will evolve. First, food will be conducted through a feeding tube placed up your nose and into your stomach. Nutrition will be supplied via this means. There is a clear fear of aspiration following intubation. Aspiration can kill you. The feeding tube will be connected to a bridle placed through the back of your septum to secure it, not comfortable but worth it.

Within days, you will then be given a swallow test. This is to prove that your throat muscles have not been damaged. The provider will instruct you to perform a series of tests to prove you can properly swallow. Following that, you will be put on a clear liquid diet for a day or two to affirm that diagnosis.

Then, finally, real food will appear! Blessed day! It has been nearly a week since you used your teeth. It may not be the best meal you have ever had, but it will be memorable.

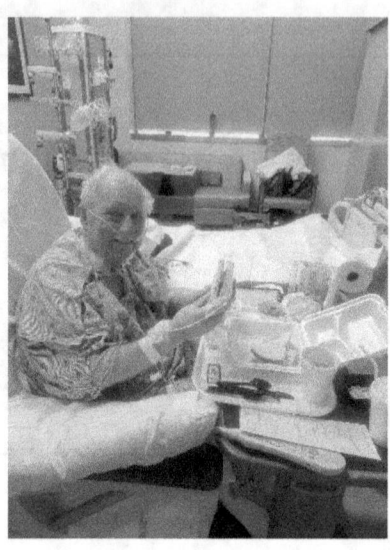

First solid Meal!

From the ICU, you will eventually be moved to a post-transplant floor in the hospital. Although still intense, you will be able to exercise more control over your own body once here. Physical fitness will begin here as well as courses on diet and medications. You will also enjoy a full bathroom with shower. Your life has changed. Embrace it.

Your stay here is again dictated by your physical condition. If you need just a little rehab, you will get out soon. If not, you stay until they are confident you are ready to be left in the hands of your caregivers. From there you will be able to leave the hospital and return to the living arrangements made for your stay near the hospital.

At this point you will be instructed in physical therapy, nutrition, and pharmacy. What you can and cannot eat and what pills you will be taking and when. This is critical. You will be taking a variety of antifungals and immune suppressants. This will continue for the rest of your life. Your body will naturally try to reject the organ, and the doctors will try to prevent that from happening. Following orders here is critical!

After the proper instructions have been administered, you will be released from the hospital to your temporary residence where you will be staying while you attend the clinic. You must be carefully watched to monitor your new organ's success.

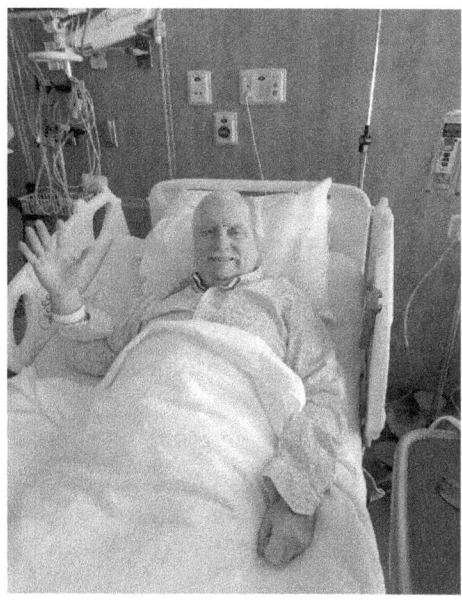

Ten days after single lung transplant surgery

Now Begins Phase Two

       Congratulations, you have received your new lung and now have a new lease on life. Use it wisely. The best way to thank your transplant team and your supporters for their hard work is to live long and prosper. You can only achieve that by FOLLOWING ORDERS! You will be given a special diet… follow it! You will be given special immune suppressive medicine…take it! The therapist will provide you with exercises…do them. You will be instructed how to protect yourself in public… act accordingly.

There are certain places you visited or functions you attended that are no longer healthy for you. Any gathering of a group of people provides risk. Sad to say, but children are especially a risk. They carry a lot of childhood diseases. Also, plants and pets must be avoided.

Below is a COVID-19 chart from the Texas Medical Association listing the probability of getting infected while in certain environments. For transplant patients, this is a good guide for informing you where you are most vulnerable to infection. Remember, your immune system is now compromised, and any infection can become serious.

       Be very careful where you go, how many people are present, and if anyone is displaying any symptoms of an infection. This applies to the rest of your life because your immune system is being suppressed to prevent rejection.

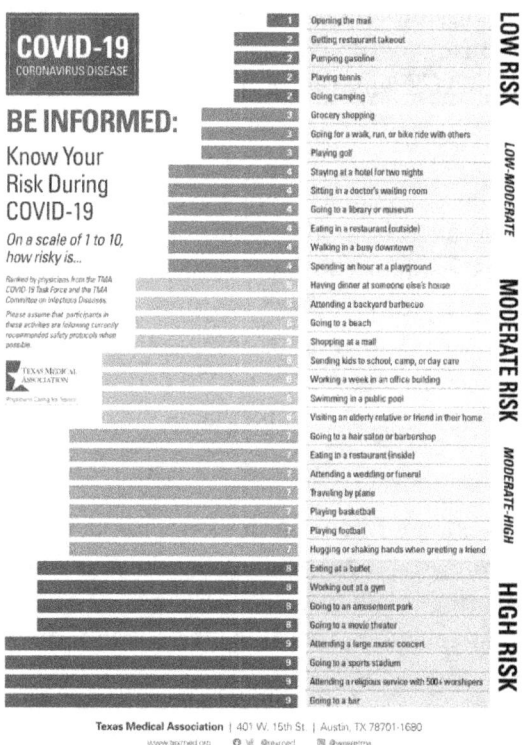

Prepare for major changes in your lifestyle. Certain foods you always enjoyed may no longer be allowed. Soft yolk eggs in particular, and raw or under-cooked food, alcohol (even wine and beer), and a variety of other items. However, a number of companies are no producing FULLY non-alcoholic beverages. My favorite is Heineken 00. This will be hard to do for some but necessary.

Before leaving the hospital you will meet with your transplant team. They will inform you about the remainder of your process. The pharmacist will meet with you to explain the medications. What they are, what they do, and how often they must be taken. The Pharmacist will present you with a weekly pill box and explain how to fill it properly.

This is very important. In fact, your life depends upon it. The pharmacist will also instruct you to never ADD any pill or SUBTRACT any pill without contacting your transplant team.

The Physical Therapist will meet and instruct you in a series of exercises you must practice in order to get your body back in shape. Remember this, you lose 10% of your strength every day you are hospitalized. If you are laid up for a few weeks or months imagine what you have lost. It takes time and special exercises to carefully rebuild yourself. But again. Walk, walk, walk, that is the best exercise for your lungs.

Next an Endocrinologist will visit. This doctor is focused on your body chemistry. The medications he/she will prescribe relate to your hormones. These pills you take may change over time as they monitor your body's chemistry.

As a result of your weekly Transplant Lab blood tests, your prescribed medicine to suppress your immune system, drugs to prevent fungal and viral infections may change. These are carefully calibrated to suit your individual needs and must be taken on a regular basis. Over time, some of these drugs may be removed, dosages changed, or others added. That is why you must stay in contact with the hospital through MyChart. Monitoring your condition and making adjustments are essential components in keeping you from rejecting your lung.

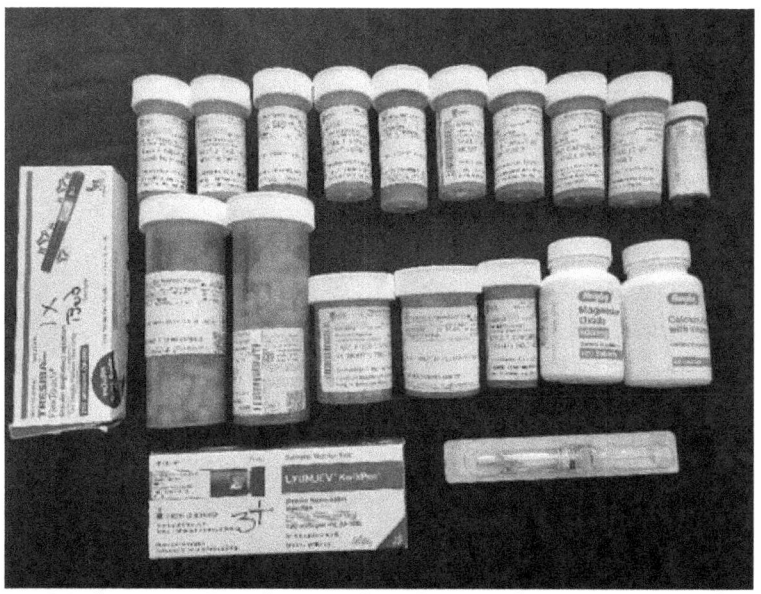

Medications I took immediately upon leaving Hospital.

Managing your pills can be confusing. In my case there were 22 different pills, two nebulizers and three shots. The pills were the most difficult to manage. There is an easy way. Take the list the pharmacist gives you and number the medicines on the paper from top to bottom. Then take the pill bottles and with a marker mark the top of each with the corresponding number. Be very careful to get this right.

The purpose for this rests in the fact that the medications have complicated names and often have several names. When your caregiver calls out a number on the list, you find the corresponding pill bottle and place the pill in its proper place. It makes things simpler.

Carefully complete the week's routine. It is best to get a weekly pill organizer with removable compartments.

This way you can take out a daily dosage and carry it with you. You cannot afford to make errors here.

This little plastic device will become the center of your existence... sad but true. You will be on immune suppressive drugs for the remainder of your life. So, get used to it and remember...it is better than the alternative!

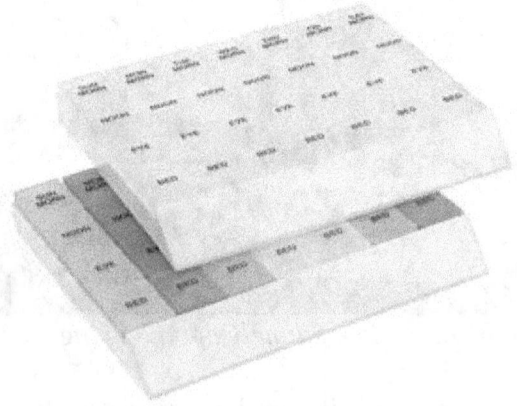

Managing medications is the single most important project you must perform. You must take the right drugs at the right time. Mistakes here can cause serious problems. These are weekly pill containers. Some are plain, others in color. I like the color ones. Each day simply pulls out which makes tracking usage easy. It also allows you to carry meds with you, so you do not miss a dose.

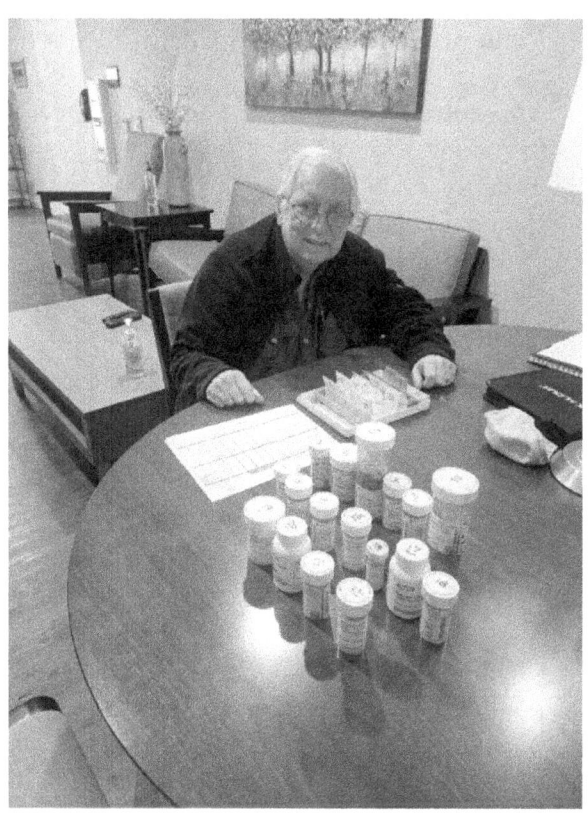

Reloading the Pillbox

The number of medicines you will take are daunting. There are so many elements needed to keep you from rejecting the lung while at the same time protecting you from opportunistic infections. Listed below are the medications prescribed for me:

Tacrolimus (Prograf) 0.5 mg – Anti-Rejection

Mycophenolate (Cellcept) 500mg-Anti-Rejection

Prednisone 10mg – Anti-Rejection

Viaganciclovir (Valcyte) – Anti-Infection (viral)

Atovaquone(Mepron)450mg–Anti-Infection (bacterial)

Itraconazole 300 mg - Anti-Fungal

Cefepime(Maximina)1g–Anti-Infection (Bacterial)

Ipratropium (Atrovent) 0.02% Nebulizer-Shortness of breath wheezing

Sodium, Chloride 3% Nebulizer-Loosening Airway Secretions

Asprin – Heart Health

Enoxaparin(Lovenox)40mgmsyringe–Anti-coagulation

Carvedilol (Coreg) 12.5 mg – Blood Pressure

Pantoprazole (Protonix) 40mg – GERD

Escitalopram (Lexpro) 5mg – Anxiety, sleep

Insulin –Dosage varies with sugar level. Medicines increase sugar.

Calcium D3 Bone Health. Some medicines cause bone weakness

Vitamin D2 - Bone Health

Vitamin C – Nutritional Enhancement

Magnesium – Electrolyte Supplements

Multivitamin – Nutritional Enhancement

Futicasone (Flonase) – Nasal Congestion

Sennosides-docusate (Senokot)–Stool Softener. Meds cause constipation

Ramelteon – Sleep

Levaquin – Antibiotic

The medication regime is not simply waking in the morning and taking a handful of pills. Were that the case it would be wonderful. Transplant patients must follow a carefully coordinated procedure each day to protect their new lung from infection and rejection In most cases this will take considerable time out of the day and living by a strict schedule.

Although tiring, it must be maintained with no exception. This is your new life, so embrace it! The alternative is organ rejection and death.

It would be wise to construct a daily chart to guide you on what to do and when. It is very easy to become confused and forgetful. This is an easy means of keeping your routine on track.

Blow illustrates the process I employ. The chart is taped on a door in easy sight as a reminder of what to do and when. As you can see, a good portion of the day one devotes to taking meds.

Morning- My routine begins in the morning when I wake up. First I must take my weight, I then take temperature, oxygen concentration, measure blood pressure, heart rate, test for sugar, take my many morning pills, and inhale two nebulizers. In some cases insulin must also be taken before breakfast.

Noon- Around noon the second process begins. Again it starts with blood pressure and sugar measurements followed by any assigned medications and insulin before lunch if required. If you are assigned a nebulizer, do it now.

Evening- In the evening again with the blood pressure, sugars, evening pills, insulin (if needed) and the nebulizer if assigned.

Bedtime- Bedtime is blood pressure, heart rate, blood sugars, prescribed pills, spirometry if required, finally oxygen at rest and oxygen after activity.

This process must be done every day with no time off! Not everyone will be on the same meds, but everyone will be on many meds and must develop a routine they can maintain. Get used to it because this routine is essential for keeping your lungs. The times when medications are taken allow some flexibility. However, some like Tacrolimus MUST be taken at twelve hour intervals.

This is the reason you want a pill box like the one shown above. Each day comes out separately. Therefore, you can take a day's worth of medications out and carry them with you if need be.

Maintaining meds is a chore. Making sure you have the meds you need on hand requires careful coordination with your pharmacy. Placing pills in pill box requires focus to get it right.   Taking meds at the proper time demands discipline. Welcome to your new world.

Every time you have lab work, the doctors review the results and adjust your meds accordingly. Thus, what you are taking today will likely change over time.

To repeat, taking meds almost becomes a full-time occupation. These pills, shots, and nebulizers must be taken at specific times. Remembering is nearly impossible, so you must devise a system for remembering. Various apps are available online to download to your phone that can alert you for scheduled medications.

Next, a dietitian will soon arrive. Food is chemistry. This person, having examined the medicines you are taking and how they are impacting your life and health, will provide you with a diet plan.   Then decisions are made about adjustments as they monitor you.   Your diet impacts your overall health during your recovery. Increasing your sugar levels due to prednisone can be expected post-surgery.

Do not be surprised if you find yourself taking insulin post-surgery.   This is due to your body's chemistry as well as the medications administered.

The Dietitian will review your chemistry and consult with the Endocrinologist. This professional will then prescribe the types of food you should eat to better benefit from what you eat. Insulin and Diabetes are common side effects of transplantation and medicines. Controlling sugar will become a serious consideration, and eating more protein and vegetables will be a focus.

For the remainder of your life you will be taking medicine to suppress your immune system. Your body will continually try to reject your new lung, it is foreign to your body and rejecting it is the purpose of your immune system. You do not have a disease that can be "cured." You have a transplant that must be maintained. Consider yourself an exotic sports car requiring constant tuning.

Initially, you will be required to attend weekly clinical tests where your condition is evaluated, and medications possibly altered. This could last three months. If all goes well, the clinical visits will lessen to twice a month, then once a month, then once every three months, till finally once a year. The schedule for this depends upon your condition post-surgery and your transplant team.

Keep in mind that the appointment times are not when you actually see the doctor or take the test. There are sometimes delays... long delays. Bring your meds, water, and something to eat. Also, have patience. The staff has a lot to do, and each patient has his/her own issues. That takes time.

You are living life on a knife's edge. It will not take much for this entire experience to go sidewise. Protect yourself which means a change in lifestyle. You owe it to a lot of people to make those necessary lifestyle changes.

You should limit your social exposure, especially in the immediate months after surgery. After that you can go about, but carefully. Visit restaurants when there is no crowd. Avoid crowded places like sports arenas or concerts. Always wear a mask. The key is to be sensible. You will always be vulnerable. I met a gentlemen at Nora's Home who had his transplant for seven years. All was well until he caught the flu. It destroyed his lung. Now he needs another transplant. The simplest infection can be devastating to you.

Your transplant team is now a permanent part of your life. Maintaining close contact and following orders will work towards your survival. It is that important. Their goal is to keep you healthy and alive. Your goal is to cooperate with them.

Expect the Unexpected

One underlying issue with a transplant, one must expect the unexpected. In my case, everything was going wonderful. Recovery was fast and my strength improving. Methodist Hospital was about to discharge me when they performed a bronchoscopy and discovered the presence of a bacterial infection.

This required an additional stay in the hospital as they monitored the situation and infused specific antibiotics to solve the problem. After six days all was well and I was discharged. Celebration day for sure.

I then went to Nora Home to begin the regular weekly health check-ups required after transplant. Over time the check-up schedule changes. This would continue for about a year. All was well… for a short while.

After about two weeks I began to have extreme chills, weakness, and shortness of breath. The first thought that comes to mind is "REJECTION." I was told to report to the Emergency Room where I was tested. The problem turned out to be COVID-19. How I got it remains a mystery because I did not leave the residency. But covid is everywhere. Nevertheless, I now had covid no matter from whence it came.

My symptoms remained mild, but I was nevertheless placed in isolation in the hospital for another six days as they administered IV anti-virials. I was then discharged again, but not allowed to return to Nora Home because of the vulnerability of the other transplant patients living there. Thankfully, the hospital placed us in a nice hotel.

The next issue was testing positive. Generally, after about 5-7 days you overcome COVID and test negative. However, it appears that those taking immune suppressors can sometimes test positive for an extended period of time. A friend with a double lung transplant contracted COVID and tested positive for three months. This creates uncertainty because of the fear of infecting others, when you do not know if you are actually contagious.

Both of these medical issues set me back quite a bit. Extra stays in the hospital, isolation, and the illness itself weakened me. Additionally, the regular routine of weekly clinical testing was stopped. I was not expecting this, but it happened. This is a lesson. Transplant patients being on immune suppressors are always vulnerable to infection. Care must be taken to prevent what could become a serious complication from simple exposure. You must always be careful and protect yourself.

That means following directions. Wear a mask when in crowds, avoid crowds as much as possible, follow directions of diet, take medications regularly, keep in contact with your Transplant Coordinator.

Again, your life has changed since the transplant. The foods you eat, the drinks you drink, and the places you go demand careful consideration. A simple infection for a normal person can be deadly for a transplant recipient.

I've learned how easy it is to become ill and how long it takes to recover. This COVID experience left me isolated for a month. Thankfully, I was not feeling that ill likely because I had the full suite of vaccinations and boosters.

I have had several people I met at Nora Home who had received lungs some time ago, but suddenly suffered a rejection. It happens quickly. A mild fever explodes to 104 degrees, breathing difficulties arise, and the next thing you know you are intubated in ICU hosting an IV of antibiotics.

You build close ties with your fellow travelers, and it hurts when one suffers a reversal. It also reacquaints one with your own vulnerabilities and the speed with which your life can change.

This is the beginning of what will hopefully be a long voyage, but one requiring significant changes in lifestyle to succeed. Your life is worth it! Always remain positive!

Additionally, every patient is different, and the medications react differently on each person. They are continually adjusting your meds based on the most recent lab work. Sometimes you do not feel well do to the many different meds and how these chemicals interact, This varies among patients.

Side effects can become a major problem and you really do not know which med is causing the issue or is it generated by a combination of drugs. You must work closely with your transplant team and inform them of any changes in your health. You cannot take any med not approved by your transplant team. If you are on something they do not know about it makes it difficult to find a solution.

Care Givers

As mentioned earlier in this work, your support team is a vital component in any transplant success. You will become totally dependent upon these loving people who must devote a significant portion of their lives to your health. This is not an easy task.

They will participate actively in every aspect of your healing. Diet, medicines, emotional support, and most importantly just general life support. In my case I am blessed with several wonderful people, my wife Margaret, my daughter Becca, and her husband Calvin. They focus totally on me. I am additionally blessed with family and friends who have been most helpful throughout.

These are the true unsung heroes. Focus is generally placed on the transplant patient, which is understandable. However, the Care Givers seldom receive the credit they deserve. They must continue doing their normal duties, must then pick-up the responsibilities of the patient, and on top of that they are expected to care for the everyday and persistent needs of the patient. It is exhausting and long-term.

My wife has stayed by my side throughout this ordeal. She never complains and is always there to do what is necessary. The level of love and commitment is beyond imagination. She has covered all the bases: for better or worse, richer or poorer, or in sickness and health. That being said, this is just what is required of a transplant Caregiver. They must put their life on hold for you.

Before surgery Margaret spent a tremendous time tending to my needs. There were many tasks I could no longer perform when on such high doses of oxygen. Once in the hospital and post-surgery, it became even more intense.

She spent every night in the ICU with me for the first several days… Sleeping on that impossible bed of nails. She was there to attend to medications, movement, getting me in and out of bed, helping with food, and every mundane need that arose she solved. Your caregiver must know that this will go on for months and can go on for the better part of a year!

Sadly, there is no way to properly prepare them for what is expected. The orientation classes devoted to Caregivers are limited in content. Yet their role is so important. Because of the intensity of effort, it is wise to have several Caregivers on call. They can easily become exhausted.

Besides them. I had many family members who likewise were present throughout to lend a hand in so many important ways. Too many to mention, but my undying thanks abound for their efforts. Just having friends send restaurant "gift cards" was a help. It takes the pressure off of the Caregiver having to prepare meals and clean up after.

The following are the accounts of Margaret, Becca, and Calvin… My wife my daughter, and her husband. This is in their own words. It is important that the support team side of the equation be mentioned so those who may care for you will know what they are getting into.

Margaret Chapman (Wife)

[My lovely wife of 50 years composed this. She has been my champion and has devoted herself to getting me well. My love for her is beyond measure. Her care for me during these years of stress is amazing. I can never thank her enough other than to express my endless love for her.]

In April 2016 we received a devastating diagnosis of pulmonary fibrosis. Next thing a pharmaceutical salesman was contacting Ron to introduce a medication for him (OFEV). He had to arrange an appointment at Ron's office, not at home. That seemed a bit strange to us. Ron did not tolerate that medication very well, and he was not comfortable with the whole situation.

Our nephew's wife is an NP with a pulmonologist in Slidell and encouraged us to make an appointment. That doctor felt it was Hypersensitivity pneumonitis (HP) and prescribed 40 mg of prednisone daily, later lowered to 10 mg. After several years of no progress an open lung biopsy was done. That only seemed to complicate matters. Ron was then transferred to a pulmonary research specialist in New Orleans. Within a period of 4 years Ron's medications included Esbriet and Tyvaso. Breathing stabilized for a while, but unfortunately Ron needed more and more oxygen for any physical movement. A 30ft. oxygen hose became his permanent appendage. He was limited in all activities but managed to exercise at least 5 days a week using YOUTUBE videos. Oxygen levels had to be raised continually when walking.

Lung transplants were not available in New Orleans, so in October 2022 our local pulmonologist referred us to Houston. We were very optimistic even though Ron's age (73) was a definite risk factor. After 5 months of traveling back and forth from home to Houston to undergo every possible test known to mankind and receiving 2 cardiac stents, Ron was denied a transplant. We all had an emotional breakdown. Total devastation!!!!! But we still had hope and refused to give up!

We were immediately referred to Houston Methodist. The original appointment was for August 2023.

Ron didn't feel like he could survive until then. Luckily, it was moved to April 4, 2023. Ron was admitted to the hospital on that day. More testing was done. Daily breathing treatments and walking was encouraged. At rest Ron was on 10 liters of oxygen and 25 liters when he walked or exerted himself. He was officially put on the transplant list on Thursday, April 20th. Monday morning at 1:14 a.m. on April 24th I received a phone call from Ron to say it was time! I tried not to panic but I was definitely moving at warp speed. A wonderful staff member from Nora's Home was nice enough to drive me to the hospital. Once there, procedures were on a roll….blood work, document signage, showers, etc.. Off he went around 4:45 a.m.. I was in the waiting room in Walter Tower. I was able to see Ron around 7:30 just before they rolled him into surgery. It was an emotional moment, yet I stayed positive and thought how wonderful it was going to be when Ron would take a breath on his own. My daughter and a dear friend were able to fly into Houston and be with me. It was very comforting to have company and support.

As the primary caregiver and wife it has been a journey. It is hard to see your loved one struggling to breathe. Daily life becomes more and more difficult. You have to stay positive and do as much as you can to simplify routines yet still make sure one functions to the max of their capabilities. They have to stay in the game. You will have good days and bad days, but you have to push ahead. The stress is difficult, but manageable. You may cry occasionally and that's okay. It helps to reduce some of the emotional pressure. Never, never give up hope. There is a light at the end of the tunnel.

Now with a new lung our job description changes. Learning the medications and the scheduling of them and new dietary restrictions is a little overwhelming but know you can do it. Just to see the transformation of your loved one is amazing. To see him without a 30ft oxygen hose is unbelievable. He has a new lease on life!

Becca Chapman (Daughter)

[My daughter and her healthcare clown partner started a business several years ago called Prescription Joy (prescriptionjoy.org). They are nationally trained therapeutic clowns who work in New Orleans Children's Hospital, Ochsner's' Hospital for Children, senior homes, St. Bernard Parish Hospital and The New Orleans Women and Children's Shelter.

Their goal is to introduce smiles into difficult situations. This is the first time she has had a close family member, her father, compromised. This gave her a different perspective on her work. This is what she posted on her website. Becca is a special young lady who possesses a heart of gold.]

THE JOURNEY

Greetings fellow Prescription Joy Community Members! Today I'd like to share a bit of my family's story with you, and how it relates to our important work.

As some of you may know, my family and I have been on a 7-month journey for my father to qualify for a lung transplant. This process has been an excruciating emotional rollercoaster of unknowns. We scheduled all our lives around tests and appointments for months. We were sometimes told by one doctor that it was very likely he would be approved for transplant, only to be told by another, just moments later, that he was too risky to operate on. It got to the point where anytime our hospital door knocked, we were sick to our stomachs. To the doctors, they were just saying "yes" or "no" to a qualification, but to us, all we hear is: "my loved one is going to live or not". The drastic emotional ups and downs were a theme park ride without the release of a cathartic scream. It took a major toll on all of us.

But we lucked out. Thanks (we believe) to the love, prayers, and support from our community, Houston Methodist took a chance. After only 5 days of being listed, Dad got a lung, *just* in time before his disease would take over completely. It is with great relief, emotional exhaustion, and hearts bursting with gratitude that we can say Dad has another chance at life. While we wade in the water of these emotions, the donor's family is still at the front of our minds. With their sacrifice in mind, Dad is determined to live for two. We have a very long road of healing ahead of us, but something that has kept us strong is JOY!

As I write this, it is easy to mention the journey as "rough and then good" just like the linear lie of healing that we all tend to believe. But the truth is, even in our worst moments, there is laughter and humor.

THE JOY

Watching my father go through this process, it is no surprise that back in 2017, Dad inspired Alex and I to start Prescription Joy in the first place. He embodies joy and cracks up the medical staff all day! So much so that nurses that worked with him on previous floors make a point to come   visit   him   in   the   ICU.

Even as my father is wheeled into transplant surgery, the height of anxiety for all of us, the nurse asked him, *"Sir, are you wearing any metal?"* to which my dad responds, *"Nah…I just took out my nipple rings."*

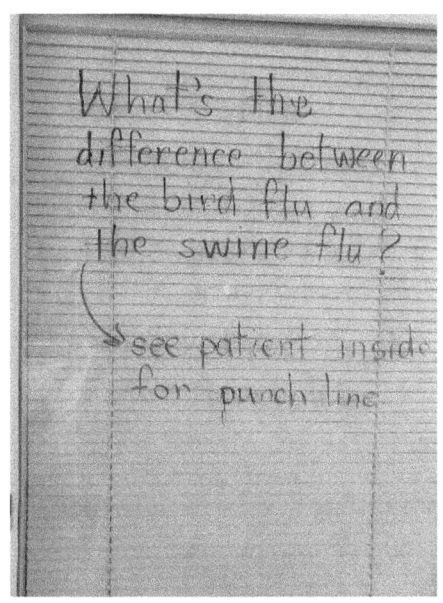

Door Joke
(Answer: Bird Flu requires a tweetment while
Swine Flu requires oinkment)

Now he is healing in the ICU, and every day we use a dry erase marker to write jokes on his window. The Medical staff have to enter his room for the punchline. So now, nurses and doctors are not just coming in with news about his body, they are entering to get the joke. This has helped heal our anxiety whenever a doctor enters our room because now, they are not the only ones with information to share :-).

It has brought unity to the halls of ICU. As mom and I exit dad's room at the end of a long day, we have nurses come up to us with hilarious urgency "OK! I have been wracking my brain! What is the punchline!?" They have expressed so many thanks to our family for the levity a simple joke can provide. As one nurse said, "It really doesn't take much, but it is important. Thank you for this."

Even though I am a Healthcare Clown whose job it is to bring joy and human connection to those in hospitals… for the first time ever I fully comprehend, from a caregiver perspective, the *NEED* and *POWER* of this work in order to survive the day to day- for patients, family members, and hospital staff. I thank my father (a natural healthcare clown) and do this work in honor of the joy he and my mother bring to   so   many.

I believe in the power of this work and have seen and felt the benefits. And this past year so did 4,039 people in our community. I am deeply honored and grateful to be in community with all of you.

Having your loved one discharged from the hospital after transplant is incredibly exciting but also terrifying for loved ones. What if we do something wrong? What if we accidentally give him something to eat that he shouldn't? What if we expose him to an illness? What if we mess up on giving insulin or administering meds? You already know what it's like to potentially lose a loved one to a disease, and now you could lose them, and it could be your fault. The stress is real. So much in your control but then so much is not at the same time.

111

Calvin Kai Ku (Becca's Husband)

[Calvin is a very special person and a close member of our family. He has become a son to me. As Director of the Medical Clown Project in San Francisco he is acutely aware of the stresses that health issues impose. He has been a true champion to us all.]

As a supporting cast, we're often faced with the question, "How can I help?" We always wish we could do more. And often what you wish you could do is out of your control. And those moments when you're simply helping to change a light bulb or helping to figure out why notifications are popping up on a phone can feel so small. But that couldn't be further from the truth.

During truly challenging periods of our lives, those little things that don't seem like much become overflowing droplets of an already overflowing bucket. Every tiny task drips beyond our capacity and continuously pokes our patience.

Recently, a friend of mine and I had a conversation about these moments. We discussed the value of "subtracting" vs "adding" to those who are emotionally and physically overwhelmed. Regardless of the size of a task, checking items off an ever-growing list will always be helpful.

Ultimately, it was tying this mantra of "subtracting" to maintaining an even keeled positivity being my relationship to our family. As much as we want to push good energy when times are down, it's important to maintain awareness and empathy along the way.

112

I'll never forget one of the most challenging moments of our journey came when we received the phone call from the first hospital denying the lung transplant. Ron and I were together, while Becca and Margaret were out of the house. The phone call lasted no more than 3 minutes. 3 minutes was all it took to crush our world. It was a tremendously sinking feeling. Stuck in our spots. Frozen in a heart crushing scene of our reality, only to be left with our thoughts of what life would be without Ron Chapman.

We weren't in a place to stay positive. We were in a place of processing. Every lingering hope by every supporting individual in our minds turned into evaporating echoes. Being denied the lung transplant literally took the air out of us.

Moments like these can be the most difficult of times, and yet they can transform into the most inspiring. We picked up the pieces and moved into action. We just got smacked across the face, but we weren't going to let it tear our sails down. Soon after, we took a tack and adjusted our heading to a new horizon that ultimately became the destination of an approved and successful lung transplant: Houston Methodist.

After witnessing and experiencing these last trying several months, seeing Ron's air shrink thinner and declining his energy, my heart is full complementing the purest tears of unequivocal joy after seeing a picture of Ron breathing fresh air in the hospital garden without oxygen tubes, and completely on his own. You often read about these kinds of stories described as "medical miracles." As a magician, this has truly been one of the most magical moments I've ever witnessed.

Couldn't be more grateful for this new lease on Ron's life, and I'm absolutely honored to be a part of this extraordinarily loving family.

Calvin Kai Ku (He/Him/His)

A Major Advance

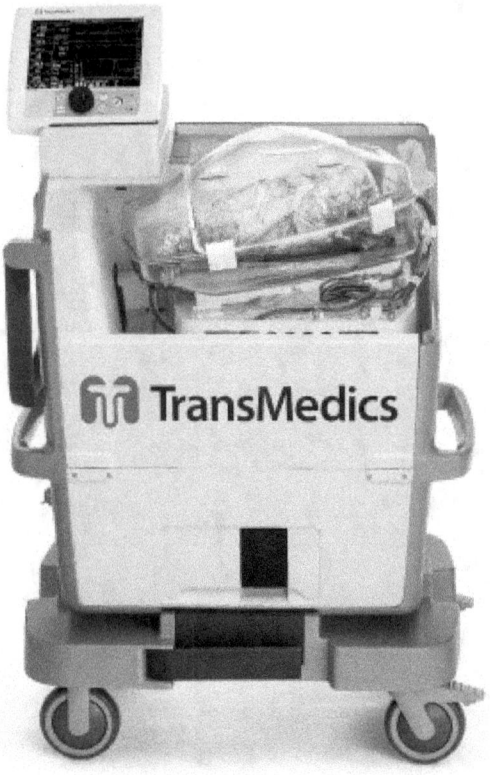

Trans Medics Lung Perfusion machine [i]

One of the main problems in the transplant world is getting the donor lung to the recipient in time. These organs are delicate and subject to damage during the journey. Traditionally, they are merely placed in an ice chest and carried to the transplant hospital. This gives the organ about six hours before serious deterioration makes it unusable.

The critical organ shortage can be somewhat mitigated through this innovative technology. Only 20% of organs offered are transplanted. That means that 80% of lungs are discorded. Additionally, the quality of lung at time of transplant contributes to the outcome that only 50% of lung transplant patients live past five years.

This is the main reason why the patient must live in close proximity to the hospital. When you get the call… you have to move fast. The fresher the lung, the better the transplant outcome.

TransMedics has solved that problem with their Organ Care System (OCS). This new technology provides transplant teams with an opportunity to save more lives. Not only does it preserve lungs for days, but indications are also that it can allow lungs that suffer some damage in the removal process to heal. It achieves this by providing a "normal" environment for the extracted lung.

This system of Ex Vivo Lung Perfusion (EVLP) was approved by the Food and Drug Administration in 2018. The EVLP system allows the lung to continue functioning as if it is still in the donors' body. Doctors can introduce steroids, antibiotics, glucose, multivitamins, and insulin into the organ will in transport.

The EVLP connects the pulmonary artery to a pump through which blood is pumped through the lung. A heater maintains body temperature. This unit takes the rush out of the organ retrieval process. It allows for careful examination of the lung, and results indicate that some lungs that have sustained damage experience a healing process.

Monitoring equipment continually tracks the lung's condition, and this allows the recovery team the ability to change the settings on the EVLP to meet immediate needs through Bluetooth technology.

According to TransMedics :*"The OCS Lung is a portable perfusion, ventilation, and monitoring system that maintains the organ at a near-physiologic state – allowing physicians to assess and improve the condition of lungs between the donor and recipient sites."*

This technological breakthrough has major implications for the Lung transplant process. As more lungs become available, they will be in better condition for transplant which extends the life expectancy of the patient.

The Transplant world is continually enjoying improvements both in surgical techniques and technology.

A Donor Story

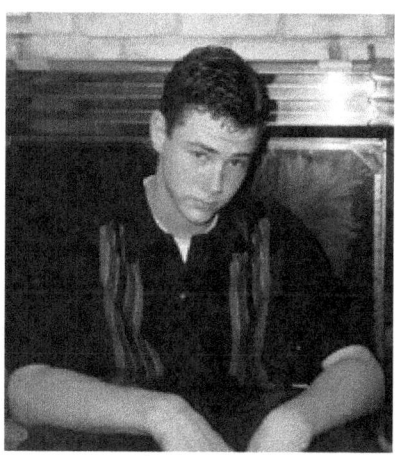

Justin Harrison

(Libby Harrison serves as a full-time volunteer with the Louisiana Organ Doar Association (LODA). She lost her son at an early age and between them they spared the lives of five individuals through organ donation. Justin set an example for us all! Since then, Libbie has devoted her life to the cause. These individuals are a blessing, especially for those who seek an organ transplant. Those of us who receive a gift organ always think of our donor. Justin's is just one story of so many,)

Wednesday morning, August 20, 1997, started just like every other school day...alarms, showers and breakfast. One small difference - I was not taking Justin to school that day. He was riding in his best friend's new pick-up truck.

I remember an enthusiastic "I love you, Mom; see ya later!" as Justin went outside. I smiled at the joy I could hear in his voice. I hope he heard my "I love you too, Buddy; have a great day!" before he closed the door. That would be my last exchange of words with my youngest child. The next time I would be by his side would be in the emergency room.

On their way home after school, at a bus stop, Justin stood up in the back of the truck to speak to friends. For some unknown reason, he tripped and fell. Emergency vehicles arrived within minutes and started life-saving procedures. In spite of their exhausting efforts, Justin was pronounced brain dead shortly after arriving at the emergency room. He was taken to the Intensive Care Unit, but we were given no hope of his survival.

As I sat there...holding his hand, begging him to wake up, pleading with God to spare my child...

I realized...Justin wasn't going home with me, his purpose on earth was complete, mine was yet to be revealed.

I did not want to take my eyes off him…his flawless face, his beautiful hair, his summer tan, his big hands that were just becoming a man's hands. It was just as important that I memorize each freckle across that perfect little nose. People were asking me questions but I couldn't speak…words seemed insignificant. My 'living' was going to be unbearable without my child.

It was incredibly hard to leave Justin's bedside when I was asked to join my husband and hospital staff in a conference room. Today, I am so thankful that I recognized the importance of this meeting. I was introduced to the Louisiana Organ Procurement Agency. When offered the opportunity of organ and tissue donation, there was no hesitation. We knew what Justin wanted.

Eleven months prior to his accident, Justin's grandfather (my father) died while waiting for a donor heart. Justin's eagerness to research donation and discover why his grandfather died made me very proud of him. At 15 years old, he was exploring a subject that most adults shy away from and yet he embraced it with youthful passion. Justin told us that if anything ever happened to him, he wanted to be a donor. His simple conclusion…if more people knew about organ donation; his PawPaw would still be alive. He said, "We gotta tell people, Momma."

So…I do. Everyday, in some way, I talk about organ and tissue donation. It's the only thing that I have left that I can do for Justin. I didn't get to see him graduate from high school, I'll never see him married nor will I ever see the grandchildren I was looking forward to meeting.

But I have met the wonderful woman who received Justin's heart. Her name is Marilyn Thorn. Our families have grown extremely close and watching her "be" with them is very comforting to us. Her family was told that she had only 48 hours to live if she didn't receive her donor heart. A few hours later they were informed of their miracle. She has had eleven years to love her children and grandchildren that she would not have had…and that makes this mother's heart smile. That heart grew inside of me for nine months and then beat inside of my beautiful son for 15 ½ years. Because of the profound limitation of words, I can't explain how comforting it is to feel his?…her?…their?... heart beating.

While I thought meeting Marilyn would be the highlight of my journey as a donor mom, more comfort was in store. This is a photo taken of Marilyn along with Sue Acaldo at our home on the 5th anniversary of Justin's death. Sue received Justin's kidney and pancreas. She was insulin dependant for 27 years and on dialysis for two years prior to transplant. Now, she is insulin and dialysis free. We spent the 10th anniversary of Justin's death celebrating life…his life and those lives he saved through donation.

Each year, we host a 'Celebration of Life' on the anniversary of Justin's death. Our family is joined by many of our friends and these two wonderful recipients, to share memories, enjoy food, games and music. We release balloons – 150 green balloons for donor awareness, 5 white balloons to represent the five lives that Justin saved and two blue balloons to represent the two people who received sight.

Through God's grace I am able to share Justin's story with you. God did indeed hear my pleas as I held Justin's hand all through that night. As I began to emerge from the 'fog' that exists during the first months of grief, I knew that I wanted to shout to the rafters that my son was a hero. Words had found their significance.

I began volunteering for the Louisiana Organ Procurement Agency (LOPA) in my new role as Donor Mom. I did not join the 'living' world until I was able to do what Justin started - telling people about organ and tissue donation. It has led to my working full-time with LOPA.

I've shared Justin's story with the media many times. Judy Bastien wrote my favorite media quote…

121

"Justin Harrison saved the lives of five people in 1997, when he was 15 years old. He did it without fanfare, through an act of quiet heroism".

My son, Justin David Harrison, is my hero.

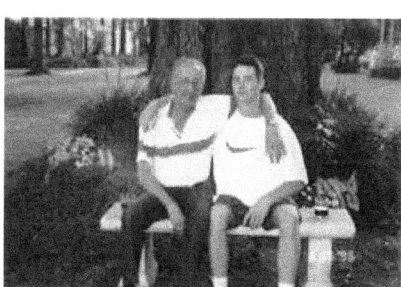 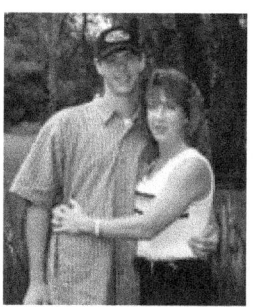

CONCLUSION

I hope this short work provides some insights into the process involved in your transplant journey. This is indeed a health issue, but you will soon realize that the life implications go far beyond your lungs.

Margaret and I were fortunate to have a friend who had a double lung transplant several years prior to my experience. He rendered invaluable insights. Nevertheless, we were not fully prepared to handle that which was about to confront us. I composed this as a helping guide to provide some insights into the process.

Remember EVERYTHING depends upon you. Your attitude, confidence, condition, and good humor are essential ingredients for a successful outcome.

1. Build a checklist for needs at home.
2. Build a checklist for needs for your remote home.
3. <u>Carefully</u> consider your budget
4. Find dedicated support. This is most important.
5. Make all necessary arrangements for : mail, checking accounts, housing.
6. If you have children, how to handle their needs.
7. Pets are a special issue.
8. Your personal physical conditioning is essential.
9. Lose weight.
10. Smile
11. Remember, the doctors, nurses and staff are there to help you. They are dedicated to the mission of

getting you well. TREAT THEM WITH THE UTMOST RESPECT!!!

`   I wish you luck on your quest because I have certainly been blessed on mine.   Love to you! Stay confident! Stay focused! Most importantly, stay in good physical condition. Your recovery depends upon it.

Remember also, at Houston Methodist Hospital you are in the very best hands. Take this from someone who has experienced a lung transplant there. I spent over a eight months in Houston with Methodist and every person I met was friendly, dedicated, and concerned about my health. They produce miracles.... I know because I am one!

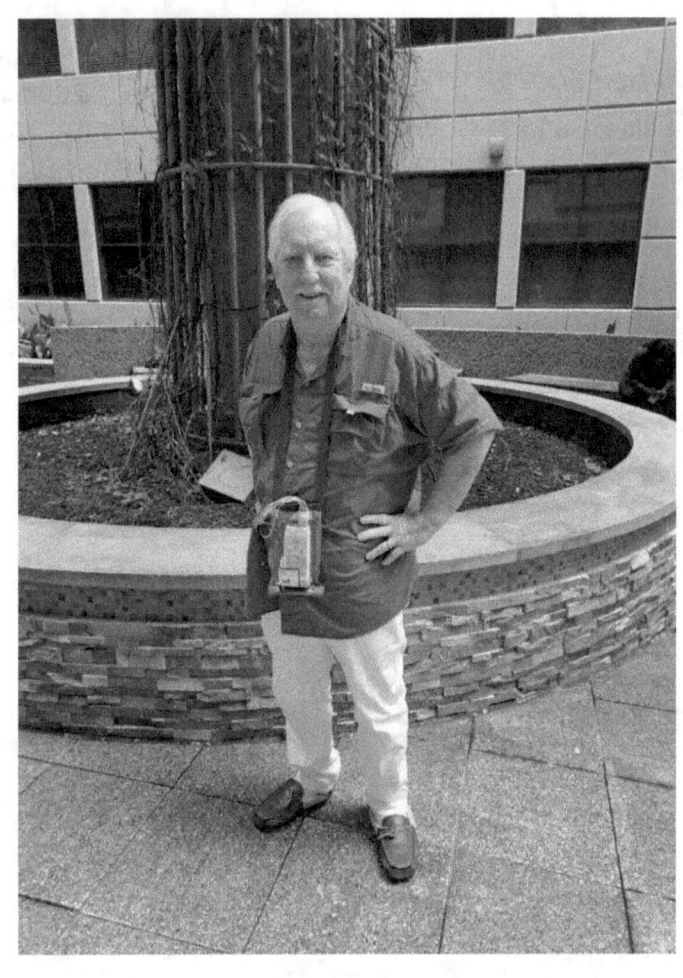

SUCCESS!!!
14 Days after Single-Lung Transplant

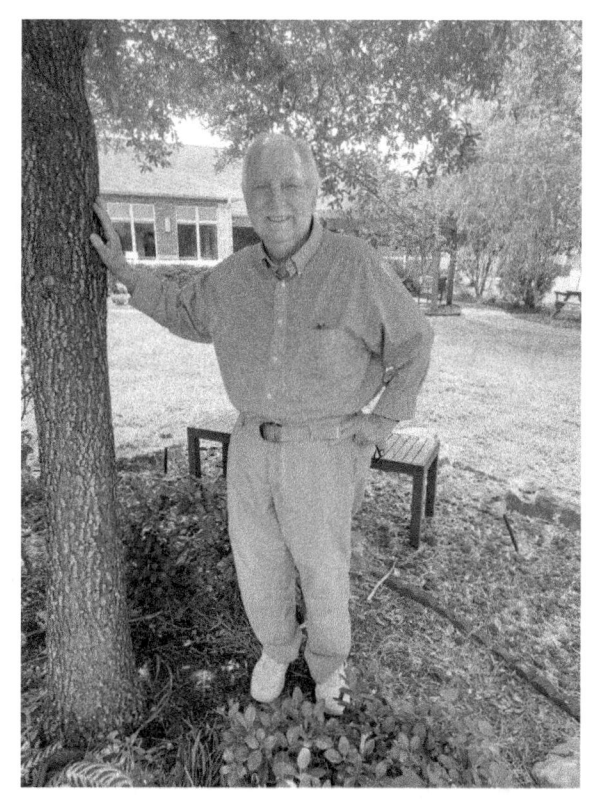

77ᵀᴴ DAY AFTER TRANSPLANT!

Epilogue

Eight Months and Counting…

It has been eight months since my April 24th single lung transplant surgery. I am only now getting home just before Thanksgiving. I was actually released early because transplant teams often require a full year of observation. This depends upon recovery. If there are complications, your stay will be longer.

It was thrilling to be able to spend Christmas at home with family, which is something I did not believe I would live to experience. I can now enjoy the thrill of my own space and association with friends on a very limited basis. It has been quite a journey.

At present I am doing fine. No indication of rejection. Trying to keep up with exercise and walking thirty minutes a day (minimum) while maintaining my medicine and vital signs drills. Those will continue for the foreseeable future. Every morning it is the same: weight, sugar, blood pressure, heart rate, and temperature. I now use insulin because the drugs appear to have raised my glucose levels. That hopefully will change as my body adjusts to the meds. You must record everything to be sent to the transplant team. Store copies. But there are no complaints, it keeps me alive.

I am also subject to monthly infusions of immunoglobulin which fortunately is being administered in my home. Doctors require infusions for six months. According to the Journal of Heart and Lung transplantation: *"The development of donor specific antibodies (DSAs) after lung transplantation has been associated with worse outcomes. Our program instituted an intensive intravenous immunoglobulin (IVIG) perioperative protocol for all sensitized patients after transplant."*

This five-hour process is much more comfortable when performed in my recliner with my books and laptop. A great convenience because I do not have to travel nor am I exposed to the hospital and infusion environment. Too many people there. Blood labs are drawn as part of this infusion process.

The blood tests are critical because they provide doctors with a record of your progress chemically. Are the immune suppressive drugs working? Should they be increased or decreased? Should other drugs be adjusted. How is my body responding to all the chemicals? Special attention must be placed on the kidneys and liver.

Presently, I take twenty-three pills per day, four insulin infusions, two nebulizers, and an oral dose of Atovaquone. This latter drug is used to prevent lung infection with Pneumocystis Carinii. This is a fungal infection that is usually present in the lungs but seldom causes problems, unless the immune system is suppressed. This was (is) a major cause of death among AIDS patients. All of these drugs are a part of my daily routine.

The two leading causes of death of lung transplant patients is CLAD and Carcinoma. CLAD (Chronic Lung Allograft Dysfunction) is defined as *"Chronic lung allograft dysfunction (CLAD) is the most common cause of mortality in lung transplant recipients after the 1st year of transplantation. CLAD has traditionally been classified into two distinct obstructive and restrictive forms:*

bronchiolitis obliterans syndrome and restrictive allograft syndrome.[ii]

This accounts for a vast majority of lung rejections, and it is wise to learn about it. The footnote below provides a good source of information.

Carcinoma is an unexpected problem. I was surprised to learn about this. Apparently, your immune system deters skin cancer under normal circumstances. However, because of immune suppression, it is a serious problem for transplants, especially among people with fair complexion. You must meet with a dermatologist nearly every four months to be checked out. Should you notice something strange, arrange for an immediate meeting. This can progress fast and metastasize.

Next month I will travel back to Houston for my scheduled "clinicals" which includes spirometry, chest x-rays, and an assortment of other tests to determine the state of my new lung. These bi-monthly visits will persist for some time. Eventually, they should occur every three to four months depending upon the results. Is my lung continuing its strong presence or is it beginning to display signs of rejection? The latter is something that continuously torments the mind.

When I left Houston Methodist I hugged Manju Johns, my transplant coordinator, and thanked her for all of the attention and efforts over the many months. She laughed and informed me that I was not going away. I will be back every few months for the rest of my life. That is one reminder of your status as a transplant recipient.

Although you feel fine, one constantly wonders if things will change. You know that rejection can happen fast.   Furthermore, the thoughts of becoming infected with some mundane disease makes one very cautious because there is nothing "mundane" when your immune system is compromised. Stay away from crowds, sick people, and always wear your mask. Your life depends upon it!

You try to function as normally as you can, however, in the back of your mind these concerns haunt. What will tomorrow bring? Nevertheless, despite these thoughts, one is thrilled to be able to live without oxygen assistance, to escape the bonds of home, and even venture into a restaurant during off-hours to enjoy dinner with family. Such normal experiences for most are exceptional thrills for me now. But I can do things, unlike when dependent on large amounts of oxygen.

As for friends, they have been so supportive, and the love expressed resonates within your heart. It is wonderful to see them and share but meet only on a limited basis. Just a few at a time.   You will still have to avoid crowds and anyone who in any way appears to be ill. Your compromised immune system dictates your life now.

When winter arrives, threats of flu, pneumonia, RSV or COVID remain strong and any of these can deliver a devastating blow. Again, with virtually no immune system, one must always be careful.   Any slip in protection may produce a difficult or perhaps even a deadly result. Also be certain to maintain vaccinations: COVID, flu, pneumonia, RSV, Shingles, etc.

As you can see, once you have received your new organ, your life will forever change. Certainly, for the better, because before transplant you were on the way out. But your new lung comes with risks and responsibilities.

You have gone through so much to get here, do not fumble now.

Lung transplants are especially difficult. Because it is the only organ open to the outside environment and is subject to a variety of assaults from illness to pollution. For that reason, the life expectancy remains far less among lung recipients than other "solid organ" transplants like liver, heart, and kidney. Therefore, those receiving a lung transplant must be far more vigilant. Additionally, many pass away from complications of some sort within five years: 80% survival within the first year, 73% three years, and 60% five years. All the more reason for vigilance. This sets out a new pattern for life. However, despite the adjustments… you are alive!!!!

Make the best of it. What matters most is that you must take every moment to enjoy the life you have been granted. Every morning when you open your eyes that day is a gift. Enjoy it and use it to its best advantage. Love those around you and cherish all relationships. Unlike most people, you realize that life has no guarantees. In some ways, this can be a blessing. It grounds one in a reality that many fail to perceive.

My journey continues as will yours. Every day is a new adventure. Yes, keeping up with meds, exercise, and vital signs can be tiring, but it is worth the results. Conditioning is important because should you be hospitalized you will need all the strength you can muster.

If you have received a transplant or listed to receive one, take heart. Never get depressed or fearful. Consider it this way. You have no alternative. Like being on a roller coaster. There will be difficulties. But you cannot get off the ride. So, throw your arms up high and scream, Weeeee!

Yes, there are a number of post-transplant issues that you must confront but never lose sight of the fact that you are alive and now have the ability to return to a near normal life. No longer are you tied to thirty feet of hose connected to an oxygen concentrator. No longer must you move about with a portable oxygen unit. You can travel, go to restaurants, meet with friends, and do things long abandoned.

For me, getting the transplant allowed me to return to teaching my college classes. Additionally, it permitted me to go back to my hobbies: stained glass, pottery, woodworking, target shooting, and re-loading. All the things I missed and had to give up because of my restrictions.

You still fact limitations like staying away from crowds, ill people, and you must wear a mask when out. But these are small prices to pay for the freedom you have earned. You are so much better off now. Focus on the positive.

Transplanting is your only hope for life. Relax and make the best of the experience.

https://pubs.rsna.org/doi/full/10.1148/ryct.2021200314#:~:text =Chronic

Transplant Centers

If you wish to see key personnel for transplant programs, use the search option "Transplant Center by Organ," and choose the specific organ.

Name ⊡	Location ⊡	Programs	Center Phone ⊡	Region ⊡
ALCH - Children's of Alabama	Birmingham, AL	Heart, Kidney, Liver	205-638-3333	3
ALUA - University of Alabama Hospital	Birmingham, AL	Heart, Heart-Lung, Kidney, Liver, Lung, Pancreas, Pancreatic Islet	866-305-5691	3
ALVA - Birmingham VA Medical Center	Birmingham, AL	Kidney	877-894-2600	3
ARBH - Baptist Medical Center	Little Rock, AR	Heart	501-202-1500	3
ARCH - Arkansas Children's Hospital	Little Rock, AR	Heart, Kidney	501-364-1100	3
ARUA - UAMS Medical Center	Little Rock, AR	Kidney, Liver, Pancreas	800-552-8026	3
AZCH - Phoenix Children's Hospital	Phoenix, AZ	Heart, Kidney, Liver	888-908-5437	5
AZGS - Banner-University Medical Center Phoenix	Phoenix, AZ	Heart, Kidney, Liver, Pancreas	800-554-1923	5
AZMC - Mayo Clinic Hospital Arizona	Phoenix, AZ	Heart, Kidney, Liver, Pancreas	480-515-6296	5
AZSJ - St. Joseph's Hospital and Medical Center	Phoenix, AZ	Kidney, Liver, Lung	602-406-3000	5
AZUA - Banner University Medical Center-Tucson	Tucson, AZ	Heart (inactive ✦), Heart-Lung (inactive ✦), Kidney, Liver, Lung, Pancreas	520-694-0111	5

CAHP - City of Hope National Medical Center (inactive ◆)	Duarte, CA	Pancreatic Islet (inactive ◆)	800-826-4673	5
CAGH - Scripps Green Hospital	La Jolla, CA	Kidney, Liver, Pancreas	858-455-9100	5
CASD - University of California San Diego Medical Center	La Jolla, CA	Heart, Heart-Lung, Kidney, Liver, Lung	619-543-6222	5
CALL - Loma Linda University Medical Center	Loma Linda, CA	Heart, Kidney, Liver, Pancreas	800-548-3790	5
CACL - Childrens Hospital Los Angeles	Los Angeles, CA	Heart, Intestine, Kidney, Liver, Pancreas	323-660-2450	5
CACS - Cedars-Sinai Medical Center	Los Angeles, CA	Heart, Heart-Lung, Kidney, Liver, Lung, Pancreas	310-423-5000	5
CAUC - University of California at Los Angeles Medical Center	Los Angeles, CA	Heart, Heart-Lung, Intestine, Kidney, Liver, Lung, Pancreas	800-825-2631	5
CAUH - Keck Hospital of USC	Los Angeles, CA	Heart, Heart-Lung, Kidney, Liver, Lung, Pancreas	888-700-5700	5
CAIM - University of California Irvine Medical Center	Orange, CA	Kidney, Pancreas	714-456-6011	5
CASJ - Saint Joseph Hospital	Orange, CA	Kidney, Pancreas	714-633-9111	5
CAPC - Lucile Salter Packard Children's Hospital at Stanford	Palo Alto, CA	Heart, Heart-Lung, Intestine, Kidney, Liver, Lung, Pancreas	650-497-8000	5
CARC - Riverside Community Hospital (inactive ◆)	Riverside, CA	Kidney (inactive ◆), Liver (inactive ◆), Pancreas (inactive ◆)	951-786-5550	5
CASM - University of California Davis Medical Center	Sacramento, CA	Heart, Kidney, Liver	916-734-2111	5
CASG - Sutter Medical Center Sacramento	Sacramento, CA	Heart	800-556-8133	5
CASH - Sharp Memorial Hospital	San Diego, CA	Heart, Kidney, Pancreas	858-939-3400	5
CACH - Rady Children's Hospital and Health Center	San Diego, CA	Heart, Kidney, Liver	858-576-1700	5

135

CAPM - California Pacific Medical Center-Van Ness Campus	San Francisco, CA	Heart, Kidney, Liver, Pancreas	877-427-6289	5
CAMB - UCSF Medical Center at Mission Bay	San Francisco, CA	Heart, Kidney, Liver	800-482-7389	5
CASF - University of California San Francisco Medical Center	San Francisco, CA	Heart, Heart-Lung, Kidney, Liver, Lung, Pancreas, Pancreatic Islet	415-353-1551	5
CASU - Stanford Health Care	Stanford, CA	Heart, Heart-Lung, Intestine, Kidney, Liver, Lung, Pancreas, Pancreatic Islet	650-723-4000	5
CALA - Harbor UCLA Medical Center	Torrance, CA	Kidney	424-306-4000	5
COUC - University of Colorado Hospital/Health Science Center	Aurora, CO	Heart, Heart-Lung, Kidney, Liver, Lung, Pancreas	720-848-2280	8
COCH - Children's Hospital Colorado	Aurora, CO	Heart, Kidney, Liver	720-777-1234	8
COPM - Centura Transplant	Denver, CO	Kidney, Liver	888-872-8891	8
COSL - Presbyterian/St Luke's Medical Center	Denver, CO	Kidney, Liver	800-758-1005	8
CTHH - Hartford Hospital	Hartford, CT	Heart, Kidney, Liver	860-972-5000	1
CTYN - Yale New Haven Hospital	New Haven, CT	Heart, Kidney, Liver	203-785-2565	1
DCCH - Children's National Medical Center	Washington, DC	Heart, Kidney	202-476-5000	2
DCGU - Medstar Georgetown Transplant Institute	Washington, DC	Intestine, Kidney, Liver, Pancreas	202-444-3700	2
DCGW - George Washington University Hospital	Washington, DC	Kidney, Liver, Pancreas	202-715-4000	2
DCWH - Washington Hospital Center	Washington, DC	Heart	202-877-7000	2

136

Code - Name	Location	Organs	Phone	
DECC - Christiana Care Health Services	Newark, DE	Kidney	866-682-6792	2
DEAI - Nemours Children's Hospital Delaware	Wilmington, DE	Heart, Kidney, Liver, Pancreas	302-651-4000	2
FLHM - Halifax Health	Daytona Beach, FL	Kidney	386-947-4650	3
FLBC - Broward Health Medical Center (inactive ◆)	Fort Lauderdale, FL	Kidney (inactive ◆), Liver (inactive ◆)	954-355-4400	3
FLUF - UF Health Shands Hospital	Gainesville, FL	Heart, Heart-Lung, Kidney, Liver, Lung, Pancreas	800-749-7424	3
FLJD - Memorial Regional Hospital/Joe DiMaggio Children's Hospital	Hollywood, FL	Heart	954-265-3437	3
FLMR - Memorial Regional Hospital	Hollywood, FL	Heart, Kidney, Pancreas	954-265-7750	3
FLSL - Mayo Clinic Hospital Florida	Jacksonville, FL	Heart, Heart-Lung, Kidney, Liver, Lung, Pancreas	877-404-6296	3
FLLM - Largo Medical Center	Largo, FL	Heart, Kidney, Liver	727-588-5728	3
FLJM - Jackson Memorial Hospital University of Miami School of Medicine	Miami, FL	Heart, Heart-Lung, Intestine, Kidney, Liver, Lung, Pancreas, Pancreatic Islet	305-355-5760	3
FLFH - AdventHealth Orlando	Orlando, FL	Heart, Heart-Lung, Kidney, Liver, Lung, Pancreas	407-303-2474	3
FLSH - Ascension Sacred Heart Pensacola	Pensacola, FL	Kidney	877-416-1600	3
FLAC - Johns Hopkins All Children's Hospital	St. Petersburg, FL	Heart	800-456-4543	3
FLTG - Tampa General Hospital	Tampa, FL	Heart, Heart-Lung, Kidney, Liver, Lung, Pancreas	800-505-7769	3
FLCC - Cleveland Clinic Florida Weston	Weston, FL	Heart, Kidney, Liver	954-689-5000	3

GAEH - Children's Healthcare of Atlanta at Egleston	Atlanta, GA	Heart, Kidney, Liver	404-785-6119	3
GAEM - Emory University Hospital	Atlanta, GA	Heart, Heart-Lung, Kidney, Liver, Lung, Pancreas, Pancreatic Islet	855-366-7989	3
GAPH - Piedmont Hospital	Atlanta, GA	Heart, Kidney, Liver, Pancreas	888-605-5888	3
GAMC - AU Medical Center, Inc.	Augusta, GA	Kidney	706-721-0211	3
HIQM - The Queen's Medical Center	Honolulu, HI	Kidney, Liver	808-538-9011	6
IAIM - Iowa Methodist Medical Center	Des Moines, IA	Kidney	888-343-4164	8
IAIV – University of Iowa Hospitals and Clinics Transplant Programs	Iowa City, IA	Heart, Heart-Lung, Kidney, Liver, Lung, Pancreas	800-777-8442	8
IAVA - The Iowa City VA Health Care System	Iowa City, IA	Kidney	319-338-0581	8
ILUC - University of Chicago Medical Center	Chicago, IL	Heart, Heart-Lung, Kidney, Liver, Lung, Pancreas, Pancreatic Islet	773-702-3000	7
ILUI - University of Illinois Medical Center	Chicago, IL	Intestine, Kidney, Liver, Pancreas, Pancreatic Islet	312-996-7000	7
ILCM - Ann & Robert H. Lurie Children's Hospital of Chicago	Chicago, IL	Heart, Intestine, Kidney, Liver, Pancreas	312-227-4030	7
ILNM - Northwestern Memorial Hospital	Chicago, IL	Heart, Heart-Lung, Kidney, Liver, Lung, Pancreas, Pancreatic Islet	312-926-2000	7
ILPL - Rush University Medical Center	Chicago, IL	Kidney, Liver, Pancreas	312-942-5000	7
ILVA - Edward Hines Jr. Veterans Administration Medical Center	Hines, IL	Kidney	844-698-2311	7

Code - Name	Location	Organs	Phone	
ILLU - Loyola University Medical Center	Maywood, IL	Heart, Heart-Lung, Kidney, Liver, Lung, Pancreas	708-216-9000	7
ILCH - Advocate Christ Medical Center	Oak Lawn, IL	Heart, Kidney	877-684-4327	7
ILSF - OSF Saint Francis Medical Center	Peoria, IL	Heart, Kidney, Pancreas	800-635-1440	7
ILMM - Springfield Memorial Hospital	Springfield, IL	Kidney	888-864-9433	7
INIM - Indiana University Health	Indianapolis, IN	Heart, Heart-Lung, Intestine, Kidney, Liver, Lung, Pancreas	800-510-2725	10
INSV - Ascension St. Vincent Hospital	Indianapolis, IN	Heart, Kidney	N/A	10
KSUK - University of Kansas Hospital	Kansas City, KS	Heart, Kidney, Liver, Pancreas	913-588-5000	8
KYUK - University of Kentucky Medical Center	Lexington, KY	Heart, Heart-Lung, Kidney, Liver, Lung, Pancreas	800-456-5287	11
KYJH - Jewish Hospital	Louisville, KY	Heart, Heart-Lung, Kidney, Liver, Lung, Pancreas	502-587-4011	11
KYKC - Norton Children's Hospital	Louisville, KY	Heart, Kidney	502-629-6000	11
LACH - Children's Hospital	New Orleans, LA	Kidney, Liver	504-899-9511	3
LAOF - Ochsner Foundation Hospital	New Orleans, LA	Heart, Heart-Lung, Kidney, Liver, Lung, Pancreas	504-842-3925	3
LATU - Tulane Medical Center	New Orleans, LA	Kidney, Liver, Pancreas	504-988-5263	3
LAWK - Willis-Knighton Medical Center	Shreveport, LA	Kidney, Liver, Pancreas	318-212-4000	3
MABI - Beth Israel Deaconess Medical Center	Boston, MA	Kidney, Liver, Pancreas	800-535-3555	1
MAMG - Massachusetts General Hospital	Boston, MA	Heart, Heart-Lung, Kidney, Liver, Lung, Pancreas, Pancreatic Islet	617-726-2000	1

MANM - Tufts Medical Center	Boston, MA	Heart, Kidney, Liver	617-636-5592	1
MAPB - Brigham and Women's Hospital	Boston, MA	Heart, Heart-Lung, Kidney, Lung, Pancreas	617-732-5500	1
MABU - Boston Medical Center	Boston, MA	Kidney	617-638-8000	1
MACH - Boston Children's Hospital	Boston, MA	Heart, Heart-Lung, Intestine, Kidney, Liver, Lung, Pancreas	617-355-6000	1
MALC - Lahey Clinic Medical Center	Burlington, MA	Kidney, Liver	781-744-2500	1
MABS - Baystate Medical Center	Springfield, MA	Kidney	413-794-2321	1
MAUM - UMass Memorial Medical Center	Worcester, MA	Kidney, Liver	800-431-5151	1
MDJH - Johns Hopkins Hospital	Baltimore, MD	Heart, Heart-Lung, Kidney, Liver, Lung, Pancreas	410-955-5000	2
MDUM - University of Maryland Medical System	Baltimore, MD	Heart, Heart-Lung, Kidney, Liver, Lung, Pancreas	410-328-6363	2
DCWR - Walter Reed National Military Medical Center at Bethesda	Bethesda, MD	Kidney	301-295-4331	2
MEMC - Maine Medical Center	Portland, ME	Kidney	207-662-0111	1
MIUM - University of Michigan Medical Center	Ann Arbor, MI	Heart, Heart-Lung, Kidney, Liver, Lung, Pancreas	734-936-4000	10
MICH - Children's Hospital of Michigan	Detroit, MI	Heart, Kidney, Liver	313-745-5437	10
MIHF - Henry Ford Hospital	Detroit, MI	Heart, Heart-Lung, Intestine, Kidney, Liver, Lung, Pancreas	313-916-2600	10
MISJ - Ascension St. John Hospital	Detroit, MI	Kidney	313-343-3047	10

140

MISM - Mercy Health Saint Mary's	Grand Rapids, MI	Kidney	616-685-5000	10
MISH - Spectrum Health	Grand Rapids, MI	Heart, Heart-Lung, Lung	866-989-7999	10
MIDV - Helen DeVos Children's Hospital	Grand Rapids, MI	Kidney	866-989-7999	10
MIBH - William Beaumont Hospital	Royal Oak, MI	Kidney, Liver	248-898-5000	10
MNAN - Abbott Northwestern Hospital	Minneapolis, MN	Heart, Kidney	612-863-4000	7
MNCM - Children's Minnesota	Minneapolis, MN	Heart	612-813-6000	7
MNHC - Hennepin County Medical Center	Minneapolis, MN	Kidney	612-873-2810	7
MNUM - University of Minnesota Medical Center, Fairview	Minneapolis, MN	Heart, Heart-Lung, Kidney, Liver, Lung, Pancreas, Pancreatic Islet	800-328-5465	7
MNMC - Mayo Clinic Hospital Minnesota	Rochester, MN	Heart, Heart-Lung, Kidney, Liver, Lung, Pancreas	507-284-2511	7
MOUM - University of Missouri Hospital and Clinics	Columbia, MO	Kidney	573-882-4141	8
MOCM - Children's Mercy Hospital	Kansas City, MO	Heart, Kidney, Liver	800-512-2168	8
MOLH - St Luke's Hospital of Kansas City	Kansas City, MO	Heart, Kidney, Liver	816-932-2000	8
MORH - Research Medical Center	Kansas City, MO	Kidney, Pancreas	816-822-8257	8
MOSL - SSM Health Saint Louis University Hospital	St. Louis, MO	Kidney, Liver, Pancreas	314-257-8000	8
MOBH - Barnes-Jewish Hospital	St. Louis, MO	Heart, Heart-Lung, Kidney, Liver, Lung, Pancreas	314-747-3000	8

MOCG - Cardinal Glennon Children's Hospital	St. Louis, MO	Heart, Kidney, Liver	314-577-5600	8
MOCH - St. Louis Children's Hospital at Washington University Medical Center	St. Louis, MO	Heart, Heart-Lung, Kidney, Liver, Lung	877-578-4449	8
MSUM - University of Mississippi Medical Center	Jackson, MS	Heart, Kidney, Liver, Pancreas	601-984-1000	3
NCMH - University of North Carolina Hospitals	Chapel Hill, NC	Heart, Heart-Lung, Kidney, Liver, Lung, Pancreas	888-263-5293	11
NCCM - Carolinas Medical Center	Charlotte, NC	Heart, Kidney, Liver, Pancreas	800-562-5752	11
NCDU - Duke University Hospital	Durham, NC	Heart, Heart-Lung, Intestine, Kidney, Liver, Lung, Pancreas	800-249-5864	11
NCEC - Vidant Medical Center	Greenville, NC	Kidney, Pancreas	252-847-4100	11
NCBG - Wake Forest Baptist Medical Center	Winston-Salem, NC	Heart, Kidney, Pancreas	336-716-2011	11
NDMC - Sanford Bismarck Medical Center	Bismarck, ND	Kidney	800-932-8758	7
NDSL - Sanford Medical Center Fargo	Fargo, ND	Kidney	701-234-2000	7
NECH - Children's Hospital & Medical Center (inactive ◆)	Omaha, NE		800-833-3100	8
NEUN - The Nebraska Medical Center	Omaha, NE	Heart, Heart-Lung, Intestine, Kidney, Liver, Lung, Pancreas	800-401-4444	8
NHDH - Mary Hitchcock Memorial Hospital	Lebanon, NH	Kidney	603-653-3931	1
NJLL - Virtua Our Lady of Lourdes Hospital	Camden, NJ	Kidney, Liver, Pancreas	856-757-3500	2
NJHK - Hackensack University Medical Center	Hackensack, NJ	Kidney, Pancreas	201-996-2000	2

NJSB - Saint Barnabas Medical Center	Livingston, NJ	Kidney, Pancreas	888-409-4707	2
NJRW - Robert Wood Johnson University Hospital	New Brunswick, NJ	Heart, Kidney, Pancreas	888-447-9584	2
NJUH - University Hospital	Newark, NJ	Liver	973-972-7218	2
NJBI - Newark Beth Israel Medical Center	Newark, NJ	Heart, Heart-Lung, Kidney	973-926-7000	2
NMAQ - University Hospital, University of New Mexico Health Sciences Center	Albuquerque, NM	Kidney	505-272-2111	5
NMPH - Presbyterian Hospital	Albuquerque, NM	Kidney, Pancreas	505-841-1234	5
NVUM - University Medical Center of Southern Nevada	Las Vegas, NV	Kidney, Pancreas	702-383-2000	5
NYAM - Albany Medical Center Hospital	Albany, NY	Kidney, Pancreas (inactive ♦)	518-262-3125	9
NYMA - Montefiore Medical Center	Bronx, NY	Heart, Heart-Lung, Kidney, Liver, Lung, Pancreas	718-920-4321	9
NYVA - James J. Peters VA Medical Center	Bronx, NY	Kidney	718-584-9000	9
NYDS - State University of New York, Downstate Medical Center	Brooklyn, NY	Kidney	718-270-1000	9
NYEC - Erie County Medical Center	Buffalo, NY	Kidney, Pancreas	716-898-3000	9
NYNS - North Shore University Hospital/Northwell Health	Manhasset, NY	Heart, Heart-Lung, Kidney, Liver, Lung	516-472-5800	9
NYNY - New York-Presbyterian Hospital/Weill Cornell Medical Center	New York, NY	Heart, Kidney, Liver, Pancreas, Pancreatic Islet	212-746-3099	9

143

NYMS - Mount Sinai Medical Center	New York, NY	Heart, Heart-Lung, Intestine, Kidney, Liver, Lung, Pancreas	212-241-6500	9
NYUC - NYU Langone Health	New York, NY	Heart, Heart-Lung, Kidney, Liver, Lung, Pancreas	212-263-7300	9
NYCP - NY Presbyterian Hospital/Columbia Univ. Medical Center	New York, NY	Heart, Heart-Lung, Intestine, Kidney, Liver, Lung, Pancreas	212-305-8110	9
NYCC - Long Island Jewish Medical Center-Cohen Children's Medical Center	Queens, NY	Heart, Kidney	855-850-8611	9
NYFL - Strong Memorial Hospital, University of Rochester Medical Center	Rochester, NY	Heart, Kidney, Liver, Pancreas	888-661-6162	9
NYSB - University Hospital of State University of New York at Stony Brook	Stony Brook, NY	Kidney	631-689-8333	9
NYUM - State University of New York Upstate Medical University	Syracuse, NY	Kidney, Pancreas (inactive ◆)	315-464-5540	9
NYWC - Westchester Medical Center	Valhalla, NY	Heart, Kidney, Liver	914-493-7000	9
OHCM - Children's Hospital Medical Center	Cincinnati, OH	Heart, Heart-Lung, Intestine, Kidney, Liver, Lung, Pancreas	800-344-2462	10
OHTC - The Christ Hospital	Cincinnati, OH	Heart, Kidney	513-585-2000	10
OHUC - University of Cincinnati Medical Center	Cincinnati, OH	Heart, Kidney, Liver, Pancreas	513-584-1000	10
OHUH - University Hospitals of Cleveland	Cleveland, OH	Heart, Heart-Lung, Kidney, Liver, Lung, Pancreas	800-844-2273	10
OHCC - The Cleveland Clinic Foundation	Cleveland, OH	Heart, Heart-Lung, Intestine, Kidney, Liver, Lung, Pancreas	216-444-0340	10
OHCH - Nationwide Children's Hospital	Columbus, OH	Heart, Heart-Lung, Kidney, Liver, Lung	614-722-2000	10

OHOU - Ohio State University Medical Center	Columbus, OH	Heart, Heart-Lung, Kidney, Liver, Lung, Pancreas, Pancreatic Islet	614-293-8000	10
OHCO - University of Toledo Medical Center	Toledo, OH	Kidney	419-383-4000	10
OKBC - Integris Baptist Medical Center	Oklahoma City, OK	Heart, Heart-Lung, Kidney, Liver, Lung, Pancreas	405-949-3349	4
OKMD - OU Medical Center	Oklahoma City, OK	Kidney, Liver, Pancreas	405-271-8000	4
OKSJ - St John Medical Center	Tulsa, OK	Kidney	918-744-2345	4
ORGS - Legacy Good Samaritan Hospital and Medical Center	Portland, OR	Kidney	877-622-8030	6
ORSV - Providence St. Vincent Medical Center	Portland, OR	Heart	503-216-2115	6
ORUO - Oregon Health and Science University	Portland, OR	Heart, Kidney, Liver, Pancreas	800-452-1369	6
ORVA - VA Portland Health Care System	Portland, OR	Kidney, Liver	800-949-1004	6
PALV - Lehigh Valley Hospital	Allentown, PA	Kidney, Pancreas	610-402-8000	2
PAGM - Geisinger Medical Center	Danville, PA	Kidney, Liver	877-821-8613	2
PAPH - UPMC Hamot	Erie, PA	Kidney	800-937-9133	2
PAHH - Pinnacle Health System at Harrisburg Hospital	Harrisburg, PA	Kidney	877-778-6110	2
PAHE - Penn State Milton S Hershey Medical Center	Hershey, PA	Heart, Kidney, Liver	800-525-5395	2
PAAE - Albert Einstein Medical Center	Philadelphia, PA	Kidney, Liver, Pancreas	215-456-7890	2

PASC - St. Christopher's Hospital for Children	Philadelphia, PA	Kidney	215-427-5000	2
PATJ - Thomas Jefferson University Hospital	Philadelphia, PA	Heart, Kidney, Liver, Pancreas	215-955-6000	2
PATU - Temple University Hospital	Philadelphia, PA	Heart, Heart-Lung, Kidney, Liver, Lung, Pancreas	215-707-2000	2
PAUP - Hospital of the University of Pennsylvania	Philadelphia, PA	Heart, Heart-Lung, Kidney, Liver, Lung, Pancreas, Pancreatic Islet	215-662-4000	2
PACP - Children's Hospital of Philadelphia	Philadelphia, PA	Heart, Heart-Lung, Kidney, Liver, Lung	800-879-2467	2
PAVA - VA Pittsburgh Healthcare System	Pittsburgh, PA	Kidney, Liver	412-360-6155	2
PAAG - Allegheny General Hospital	Pittsburgh, PA	Heart, Kidney, Liver, Pancreas	412-359-3131	2
PACH - UPMC Children's Hospital of Pittsburgh	Pittsburgh, PA	Heart, Heart-Lung, Intestine, Kidney, Liver, Lung, Pancreas	412-692-5325	2
PAPT - University of Pittsburgh Medical Center	Pittsburgh, PA	Heart, Heart-Lung, Intestine, Kidney, Liver, Lung, Pancreas	877-640-6746	2
PALH - The Lankenau Hospital (inactive ✦)	Wynnewood, PA	Kidney (inactive ✦)	484-476-2000	2
PRSJ - Auxilio Mutuo Hospital	Hato Rey, PR	Kidney, Liver, Pancreas	787-758-2000	3
PRCC - Cardiovascular Center of Puerto Rico and the Caribbean	San Juan, PR	Heart	787-754-8500	3
RIRH - Rhode Island Hospital	Providence, RI	Kidney	401-444-4000	1
SCCH - MUSC Children's Hospital	Charleston, SC	Heart	843-792-5097	11
SCMU - Medical University of South Carolina	Charleston, SC	Heart, Heart-Lung, Kidney, Liver, Lung, Pancreas	843-792-5097	11

146

SCPG - Prisma Health Greenville Memorial Hospital	Greenville, SC	Kidney	864-455-7000	11
SCLA - MUSC Lancaster	Lancaster, SC	Kidney	803-286-1481	11
SDMK - Avera McKennan Hospital	Sioux Falls, SD	Kidney, Pancreas	605-322-7350	7
SDSV - Sanford Health/USD Medical Center	Sioux Falls, SD	Kidney	605-328-9290	7
TNEM - Erlanger Medical Center	Chattanooga, TN	Kidney	423-778-7000	11
TNUK - University of Tennessee Medical Center at Knoxville	Knoxville, TN	Kidney	865-305-9000	11
TNLB - Le Bonheur Children's Medical Center	Memphis, TN	Heart, Kidney, Liver	901-287-5437	11
TNMH - Methodist University Hospital	Memphis, TN	Kidney, Liver, Pancreas	866-805-7710	11
TNBM - Baptist Memorial Hospital	Memphis, TN	Heart	800-422-7847	11
TNST - Saint Thomas Hospital	Nashville, TN	Heart, Kidney	615-222-2111	11
TNVU - Vanderbilt University Medical Center	Nashville, TN	Heart, Heart-Lung, Kidney, Liver, Lung, Pancreas	615-936-0388	11
TXCT - Seton Medical Center Austin	Austin, TX	Heart	877-377-3866	4
TXDL - Dell Children's Medical Center	Austin, TX	Heart, Kidney (inactive ◆)	512-324-5942	4
TXDM - North Austin Medical Center	Austin, TX	Kidney	512-901-1000	4
TXDS - Dell Seton Medical Center at The University of Texas at Austin	Austin, TX	Kidney, Pancreas	512-324-7000	4

TXDC - Driscoll Children's Hospital	Corpus Christi, TX	Kidney	800-324-5683	4
TXHD - Medical City Dallas Hospital	Dallas, TX	Heart, Kidney, Pancreas	972-566-7199	4
TXCM - Children's Medical Center of Dallas	Dallas, TX	Heart, Kidney, Liver, Pancreas	214-456-7000	4
TXMC - Methodist Dallas Medical Center	Dallas, TX	Kidney, Liver, Pancreas	214-947-1800	4
TXPM - Parkland Health and Hospital System	Dallas, TX	Kidney	214-590-8000	4
TXSP - UT Southwestern Medical Center/William P. Clements Jr. University Hospital	Dallas, TX	Heart, Heart-Lung, Kidney, Liver, Lung	214-633-5555	4
TXTX - Baylor University Medical Center	Dallas, TX	Heart, Heart-Lung, Kidney, Liver, Lung, Pancreas, Pancreatic Islet	214-820-2050	4
TXDR - Doctor's Hospital at Renaissance	Edinburg, TX	Kidney	956-362-8677	4
TXLP - Las Palmas Medical Center	El Paso, TX	Kidney	915-264-7800	4
TXPL - Medical City Fort Worth	Fort Worth, TX	Kidney, Pancreas	817-834-8500	4
TXFW - Texas Health Harris Methodist Fort Worth Hospital	Fort Worth, TX	Kidney	800-411-2443	4
TXCF - Cook Children's Medical Center	Fort Worth, TX	Kidney	682-885-4000	4
TXAS - Baylor Scott and White All Saints Medical Center-Fort Worth	Fort Worth, TX	Kidney, Liver, Pancreas, Pancreatic Islet	800-774-2487	4
TXJS - University of Texas Medical Branch at Galveston	Galveston, TX	Heart, Kidney, Pancreas	409-772-1011	4

TXMH - Houston Methodist Hospital	Houston, TX	Heart, Heart-Lung, Kidney, Liver, Lung, Pancreas	713-394-6000	4
TXVA - Michael E. DeBakey VA Medical Center	Houston, TX	Heart, Kidney, Liver	800-553-2278	4
TXHH - Memorial Hermann Hospital, University of Texas at Houston	Houston, TX	Heart, Heart-Lung, Kidney, Liver, Lung, Pancreas	713-704-4000	4
TXHI - CHI St. Luke's Health Baylor College of Medicine Medical Center	Houston, TX	Heart, Heart-Lung, Kidney, Liver, Lung	713-785-8537	4
TXTC - Texas Children's Hospital	Houston, TX	Heart, Heart-Lung, Kidney, Liver, Lung	832-824-1000	4
TXUC - University Children's Health	San Antonio, TX	Kidney, Liver	888-336-9633	4
TXHS - Methodist Specialty and Transplant Hospital	San Antonio, TX	Heart, Heart-Lung (inactive ♦), Kidney, Liver, Pancreas	800-888-0402	4
TXBC - University Hospital, University of Texas Health Science Center	San Antonio, TX	Kidney, Liver, Lung	210-358-4000	4
TXSW - Scott and White Memorial Hospital	Temple, TX	Heart, Kidney, Pancreas	254-724-2111	4
UTLD - Intermountain Medical Center	Murray, UT	Heart, Kidney, Liver, Pancreas	866-439-0480	5
UTMC - University of Utah Medical Center	Salt Lake City, UT	Heart, Heart-Lung, Kidney, Liver, Lung, Pancreas	801-581-2121	5
UTPC - Primary Children's Hospital	Salt Lake City, UT	Heart, Kidney, Liver	800-909-7262	5
VAUV - University of Virginia Health Sciences Center	Charlottesville, VA	Heart, Heart-Lung, Kidney, Liver, Lung, Pancreas, Pancreatic Islet	434-924-0211	11
VAFH - Inova Fairfax Hospital	Falls Church, VA	Heart, Heart-Lung, Kidney, Lung, Pancreas	703-776-4001	2

VACH - Children's Hospital of the King's Daughters	Norfolk, VA	Kidney	757-668-7000	11
VANG - Sentara Norfolk General Hospital	Norfolk, VA	Heart, Kidney, Pancreas	757-388-3000	11
VAHD - Henrico Doctors' Hospital	Richmond, VA	Kidney	804-289-4500	11
VAMC - VCU Health System Authority, VCUMC	Richmond, VA	Heart, Kidney, Liver, Pancreas, Pancreatic Islet	804-828-9000	11
VAMV - Hunter Holmes McGuire Veterans Administration Medical Center	Richmond, VA	Heart	804-675-5000	11
VTMC - The University of Vermont Medical Center	Burlington, VT	Kidney	802-656-2345	9
WACH - Seattle Children's Hospital	Seattle, WA	Heart, Intestine (inactive ✦), Kidney, Liver, Pancreas	866-987-2000	6
WASM - Swedish Medical Center	Seattle, WA	Kidney, Liver, Pancreas	206-386-6000	6
WAUW - University of Washington Medical Center	Seattle, WA	Heart, Heart-Lung, Intestine (inactive ✦), Kidney, Liver, Lung, Pancreas	866-894-3278	6
WAVM - Virginia Mason Medical Center	Seattle, WA	Kidney, Pancreas	888-862-2737	6
WASH - Providence Sacred Heart Medical Center & Children's Hospital	Spokane, WA	Heart, Kidney, Pancreas (inactive ✦)	800-667-0502	6
WIUW - University of Wisconsin Hospital and Clinics	Madison, WI	Heart, Heart-Lung, Kidney, Liver, Lung, Pancreas	608-263-6400	7
WICH - Children's Hospital of Wisconsin	Milwaukee, WI	Heart, Kidney	877-266-8989	7
WISE - Froedtert Memorial Lutheran Hospital	Milwaukee, WI	Heart, Heart-Lung, Kidney, Liver, Lung	800-805-4700	7

WISL - <u>Aurora St. Luke's Medical Center</u>	Milwaukee, WI	Heart, Kidney, Liver, Pancreas	888-863-5502	7
WVCA - <u>Charleston Area Medical Center</u>	Charleston, WV	Kidney	304-388-7823	2

NOTES

[1] https://www.ncbi.nlm.nih.gov/pmc/articles/PMC6783715/